Diego De Leo

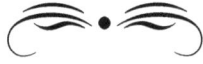

TURNING POINTS

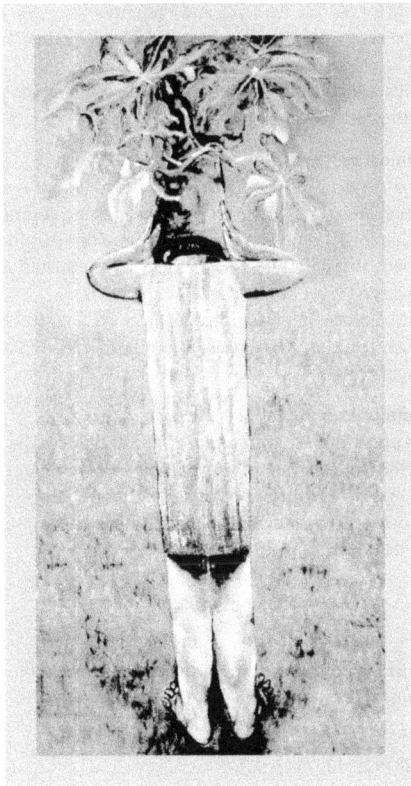

An Extraordinary Journey
Into the Suicidal Mind

First published in 2010
Australian Academic Press
32 Jeays Street
Bowen Hills Qld 4006
Australia
www.australianacademicpress.com.au

All author royalties from *Turning Points* will be donated to the following non-profit organisations:
1. Australian Institute for Suicide Research and Prevention
2. De Leo Fund (International), which supports suicide researchers from developing countries.
3. De Leo Fund Onlus, which supports clinical services for bereaved persons following suicide or traumatic death.

National Library of Australia Cataloguing-in-Publication entry

Author:	De Leo, Diego, 1951-
Title:	Turning points : an extraordinary journey into the suicidal mind / Diego De Leo.
Edition:	1st ed.
ISBN:	9781921513374 (pbk.)
Subjects:	Suicide--Psychological aspects. Suicide victims--Psychology.
Dewey Number:	616.858445

The cover illustration is a painting by Zivko Marusic, entitled 'Albero tagliato rigenerato', which means 'cut tree, regenerated'.

I congratulate Professor Diego De Leo on his professionalism and dedication in bringing this extraordinary collection of moving stories together. I'm proud to endorse this book, which I consider an important addition to the literature on loss, grief, hope and generosity of spirit. Diego, in his life and work, has always drawn on these elements personally, professionally and with great eloquence. I highly recommend this book for families, parents, young people and health practitioners.

Leonie Young, CEO, *beyondblue*

For as long as recorded history suicide has been part of society, yet it is still not well understood and is shrouded in folklore. To realise a more compassionate world it is essential for all of us to become more informed about why people think about and attempt suicide and what helps us hold on to life and living. These heart-rending personal accounts take us one step closer to a greater understanding of this complex, human struggle.

Dawn O'Neil, CEO, Lifeline Australia

This book features compelling vivid stories by those who have returned from the brink of eternity. Accompanied by reflective commentaries from eminent suicidologist Diego De Leo, they offer a remarkable illumination of the condition of suicidal people. Their testimonies celebrate both the lives of survivors and a distinguished researcher whose capacity to listen deeply is the hallmark of the finest clinical practice.

Associate Professor **Michael Dudley,**
Chair, Suicide Prevention Australia

This powerful and very moving collection of stories has much we can learn from. We learn that people can grow from the depths of despair to regain a life worth living, that if we were to provide treatment early for mental illness then lives could be saved, and that if we support families who are bereaved then we can make a real difference.

Barbara Hocking,
Executive Director, SANE Australia

To Nicola and Vittorio, and all
others who are always with us
but cannot be hugged anymore

Green Shoots of Hope

Julianne Schultz

e are all the product of events and experiences that are beyond our control. The way we respond to them is more within our control, but that too can be fraught and subject to factors we could not anticipate or plan for.

Often when we look at the work and achievements of people who have made a major contribution we see what they have contributed, how they have changed our way of seeing and thinking, how their dedication and insight has made a difference.

We rarely get an insight into what set them on this journey, the moment that triggered a lifetime of research and study, the complex emotions that sit at the base of a public and intellectual life.

This is understandable, these are the things most of us like to keep private, we don't want to bore others with intimate details of our own journey. In general, we are more interested in and tend to celebrate the destination rather than the path that got us there.

The great value of this book, and indeed of Diego de Leo's work more broadly, is that it focuses on the journey, not just the end. For someone who deals with death every day this is particularly important, and as he tells in chapter 1, this approach is the product of his own experience.

It was the death of a colleague that triggered the trajectory of Diego's career. His sense of loss and inadequacy in failing to anticipate or understand the suicide of another brilliant young doctor set him on a path that has resulted in his deep knowledge of suicide, and has provided him with the tools to provide support and comfort to many contemplating taking their own lives, and their families and friends. This youthful experience not only sowed the seeds for a fascinating and rich intellectual life, but has enabled him to see the tangible benefits of this work in the lives of others.

I was privileged to come across Diego's work and writing when I was preparing an edition of *Griffith REVIEW* entitled 'Staying Alive'. That edition explored many of the big issues of life and death, from the successful Australian approach to public policy management of the HIV-Aids pandemic and the less successful approach to ensuring Indigenous health and longevity, to the challenging personal and legal issues of euthanasia, to the peace for the dying and their families that can come from sensitive, emotionally rich palliative care.

Diego's work in suicide prevention offered another per-spective, one which I had not heard of before — one that was hopeful and suggested that there could be a light at the end of even the darkest tunnel. As he told me about his patients who had come back from the brink of thinking that life was not worth living, I realised yet again that the human spirit is a remarkably resilient thing. That out of the darkest earth of despair green shoots could sprout.

Many of us have been touched by the tragedy of suicide, it is as he says the 'the worst of all human tragedies. Not only does it often represent the epilogue to unbearable suffering for the person who commits it, but also it may be the source of incredible pain for those who survive the loss'.

That part of the suicide story is well known. What is much less well known is what can happen to those who attempt, but fortunately fail, to take their lives. As this book demonstrates, this can provide an unexpected opportunity to start again. No-one would wish this cathartic journey on another, it is a gamble with ridiculous odds, but it is remarkably reaffirming to read these stories and realise that despite a sense of insurmountable hopelessness, all is not lost, life can go on, it can get better when we take control and accept ownership and treatment of our own problems and frailties.

As Diego knows better than most from his work and in the tragedy that has touched his own life, 'Most people, at some stage in their lives, encounter difficult circumstances or personal crises. One in six considers suicide as a possible option in such situations. Fortunately, the vast majority of people overcome the difficulties and control self-destructive impulses. Death is just the medium to avoid the continuation of the unbearable'.

But sometimes with time, treatment and love the unbearable can become bearable — there are green shoots waiting to germinate.

As the debate about euthanasia attests, this is a very complex, emotionally, spiritually and medically fraught discussion, one that will not be readily or easily resolved. But in collecting the stories of people who have come close to death, survived and continued to live productive, meaningful and hopeful lives, we have a beacon for the darkest moments.

Diego de Leo is a scholar and public intellectual of extraordinary capacity, who has used his personal experiences to inform a lifetime of work, and provide comfort and inspiration to us all.

Dr Julianne Schultz AM is the founding editor of *Griffith REVIEW.*

Contents

Part ONE

Diego's story

~≈≈⌣

ONE

Studying Suicidal Behaviours
Diego's Story

*I*n 1981, at the age of 29, I was in my last year as a registrar in psychiatry at the University of Padua in northern Italy.
As was customary in that school at the time, I was assigned —
for the first time — a newly appointed registrar, four years
younger than me. My role was to guide him in his clinical and
research developments. A more senior staff member was in
charge of supervising both of us.

In those days, the Department of Psychiatry was characterised by the psychoanalytical approach, and we were strongly
encouraged to become fully immersed in the theories of Freud
and his followers. However, my inclination was towards other
theories. From a very young age, I'd been intrigued by the
mind–body interaction, and I wanted to understand how the
brain (cells, nerves and the like) could be the origin of feelings
and thoughts. The possibility that negative emotions, or
symptoms like depression and anxiety, may provoke alterations
and diseases in the body fascinated me. I hoped that my choice
of psychiatry could help clarify these issues.

In any case, with some reluctance (called 'resistance' among
the psychoanalytic adepts) I started my psychoanalytical
therapy/training. I must admit that, more than an expression

of an authentic credo, it was a way of being accepted by the local psychiatric environment.

The young registrar was soon revealed to be very nice: intelligent and witty, always cheerful and ready to joke about everything, he nonetheless seemed seriously motivated to become a researcher and shared my passion for the mind–body interface. Consequently, as two clandestine researchers — and as far away as we could get from our supervisor — we started a 'forbidden' study of psychosomatics. At that time I had the firm conviction that certain people, characterised by a particular personality type and particular behaviours, were more exposed than others to the risk of heart attack. The theories of an American scientist, Professor David Jenkins, appealed to me. He thought that there were two main patterns of behaviour, Types 'A' and 'B', which were associated with totally different predispositions to cardiac diseases: Type A the assertive, hard-driving, ambitious and aggressive, and Type B the relaxed, tolerant, contemplative and spiritually oriented. Intuitively, Types A were at risk, while Types B were relatively protected. In almost covert contact with Professor Jenkins, we started to study a population of heart attack survivors to verify whether their personalities and behaviours were in line with our expectations.

My young co-worker was the son of a well-known professor in the same faculty of medicine at our university. The idea of potentially being under special scrutiny because of this did not affect my audacity. On the contrary, the presence of an important family name fortified my determination in that very innocuous conspiracy against the psychoanalytical establishment. We know that universities should be flag-bearers of intellectual freedom, but we also know that this is rarely so. And even if our aim was merely to study something that interested us, the consequences of our deviant behaviour were to be feared. To reduce their impact, we also started some studies on psychoanalytical topics.

Of course, the cover-up lasted only *l'espace d'un matin*. We were not expelled (that would have been too much), but the strong antibodies the environment generated against us soon became very significant. We were not made part of mainstream initiatives, and we obtained only limited access to funding opportunities. Heresy has a price, as history teaches, and I learned later that our department was certainly not the only institution in which psychoanalysis was professed as a religious doctrine rather than treated as a science. Anyhow, that ridiculous discrimination cemented our cooperation, and transformed us from accomplices into friends.

About three years after the beginning of our research on Type A behaviour patterns, our first paper appeared in a reputable medical journal, and other research followed over the next two years. As soon as I received a copy of the publication, I called my friend to invite him for a toast in celebration of our small achievement. On the phone he said that he was very busy, but he would try to make time for a meeting over the weekend.

I didn't hear from him. I paid no particular attention to that; he often disappeared for days with his girlfriend of the moment (he seemed to be a prodigious *tombeur de femmes*) and, without a formal contract with the department, he normally came only to see me and discuss our research projects. But two weeks without communication had never occurred before.

My concern did not last too long. One morning, Anna — a colleague with whom I shared a room at the institute — did not greet me with the usual 'Ciao'. Instead she said: 'Have you heard?'

'Heard what?' I replied without particular apprehension.

'What your young friend has done: he has killed himself! Didn't you realise how much that guy was suffering?'

In pronouncing the verdict sanctioning my perennial incompetence, Anna passed to me a copy of the local newspaper. A two-column article explained that my friend had shot himself at dawn with his father's pistol in a bushy area of the hills surrounding Padua. Apparently he had walked for quite a while before reaching the place.

I could not believe it. It must have been someone else, maybe with the same name and profession, but not him. My eyes full of tears, I read and reread the article. I refused to believe that my friend — my splendid, intelligent, brilliant friend — was the same person who had carried out this insanity. And, God, I did not see him suffering at all! How could Anna say something like that?

Anna, who had continued to stare at me while I was frantically searching backwards in my memory files for some hints in justification of the senseless act, did her best to demolish me.

'What sort of psychiatrist are you going to be, if you are not even able to understand the people around you?'

More than 25 years later, I still distinctly remember Anna's words. Indeed, I remember everything of that moment: the colour of the day, the dress she was wearing, the smell of Toscano cigars in the room (we smoked in hospitals then), and the newspaper over my desk. And, of course, Anna's accusatory eyes.

The family of my young colleague and friend never sought any contact with me. They held a private funeral and never replied to my long, passionate letter. This made everything even more traumatic and painful. His death remains forever a mystery to me; the silence from the family was absolute. A few rumours suggested that he had been abusing drugs (cocaine? amphetamines?) or had been sick. But sick from what? He looked to me absolutely normal — and certainly happier than me, to be honest.

*   *   *

Suicide is the worst of all human tragedies. Not only does it often represent the epilogue to unbearable suffering for the person who commits it, but also it may be the source of incredible pain for those who survive the loss. It may constitute a life-changing experience. The most common reactions are disbelief, guilt, anger, anxiety and depression, but survivors may also experience fear of becoming crazy, fear of being predestined to suicide, and being stigmatised forever. Or they may simply feel that, without the lost person, life is meaningless, thus consider suicide — their own — as a possible way out. This psychological suffering marks the existence of those left behind and, with different degrees of intensity, may accompany them throughout their lives.

These conditions are far from rare. Based on World Health Organization data there were approximately 880,000 cases worldwide in 2003. It has been calculated that every year an average of four-and-a-half million individuals have their lives deeply affected by a suicide. Given the fact that the scars from the event are present for life, the number of people who continue to live with the consequences of a suicide is enormous. Most struggle in search of explanations, something that may help them to recompose a more peaceful picture inside their hearts.

Since my friend's unexpected suicide (a turning point for me), my life has been dedicated to studying and preventing suicidal behaviours. Having become a known expert, many people contact me in an effort to understand what has happened. Parents who approach me after the suicide of children usually bring diaries, drawings and possessions belonging to the deceased, and sometimes a suicide note. They hope I might identify from this material useful elements to provide sensible explanations — why he (far more often than she) did it. When I ask whether there was any clue that may have predicted what happened, the answer is always more or less the same: 'Nobody could have expected anything like that!'

Attending one of my first international conferences on suicidal behaviour in the United States many years ago, I was struck by the logo of the congress: a big ear. Organisers and registered attendees were wearing a badge with the same symbol. Since the location was a big hotel where different exhibitions/conferences could be held simultaneously, I feared I was mistakenly addressing myself to an otologists' convention. Finally, I could read what was written below the big ear: 'I have the ear' — meaning I know how to listen, hence I may understand.

This is one of the critical aspects of suicide prevention. How many people really know how to listen, and how many are willing to do so? Is it possible that many parents do not 'have the ear', do not listen to their children? It seems that in a number of cases this is what occurs. Those parents were unable to pick up danger signals that could have been important warning signs. They did not pay enough attention to what was happening in the troubled lives of their sons and daughters, who shut the door on their young lives, leaving the parents, shocked and traumatised, to exchange accusations with each other and to look for ethereal culprits in contemporary society, empty of any value, materialistic, cynical. The family that brings up, educates, gives support and shelter to a child is the prime form of society for the developing individual. It is better to look inside first, and then eventually outside.

Obviously, society has its own responsibilities. This is undeniable. All researchers are aware of the negative influence of factors like unemployment, economic recession, individualism, separation and divorce, alcohol and drug abuse, criminal behaviour, secularisation, and so on. All these factors (and others) are important, but they merely provide what are called 'epidemiological profiles' of suicidal people, which means that they simply aggregate those elements found most commonly in individuals who kill themselves.

But you cannot report this to the grieving families. They don't care about the increased participation of women in the labour force, or the lack of spirituality in society. They want specific, personalised answers. They want to understand why it happened, and why to them — the parents of a non-psychiatrically disturbed child.

This is another crucial point in suicide prevention. In fact, if a great number of suicides are undoubtedly affected by a psychiatric condition at the time of their death, there are also many in which there is no evidence of such an illness. Of course, these situations embarrass us most, because it would be very reassuring to think that suicide happens only to psychiatric patients. This way of considering suicide is unfortunate but deeply rooted. The Church had a role, permitting burial in holy soils only those suicide victims who were *non compos mentis* (i.e., mentally insane). This attitude has changed only recently. I am not saying that we don't have to fight psychiatric diseases to prevent suicide, but this would probably solve only a part of the problem. Suicide is a very complex phenomenon ('The only serious philosophical problem', in the words of the French philosopher Albert Camus), and to be properly addressed it requires multiple remedies. Maybe more appreciable modifications in suicide rates would be achievable through social and cultural changes.

Most people, at some stage in their lives, encounter difficult circumstances or personal crises. One in six considers suicide as a possible option in such situations. Fortunately, the vast majority of people overcome the difficulties and control self-destructive impulses. However, the very fact that suicidal ideation is so widespread in the community underscores the preoccupation about death that characterises our society, which generally reacts with the denial.

There have always been people who wished to end their lives. A *Dialogue of a Misanthrope with His Own Soul*, describing quite eloquently a chain of suicide ideations, is attributed to an Egyptian scribe more than 4000 years ago. With very few exceptions suicide is present in every culture. This may look incredible, because there is nothing more important than life. Those individuals, who even in interminable pain, or suffering unbearable tortures, profound humiliations, or facing imminent death, tenaciously resist it, demonstrate this. However, there are people who decide to put an end to their lives. These people must perceive their existence as so frustrating, unrewarding and meaningless that they are induced to *sua manu cadere* (literally to fall by their own hand, the typical Latin expression that identified the act of self-killing in the ancient Rome; the term 'suicide' appeared in the literature only in the seventeenth century).

Consequently, instead of waiting for the natural course of life to end, they decide to prematurely interrupt their existence. In most cases their reasoning is flawed, the product of an emotionally troubled mind. If we want to avoid the irreparable, we need to interfere with this process as soon as possible. Very frequently, the subjects themselves perform this operation; sometimes their proxies (a partner or friends) intervene; on other occasions general practitioners or counsellors do so. Crisis intervention is a key concept in suicide prevention: it assumes that acute suicidality lasts for a maximum of several hours, or a few days. Once the crisis is overcome, subjects may regain control of their lives.

Unfortunately, sometimes nobody intervenes — despite the fact that most suicidal people communicate, more or less directly, their intention to die. Certain people do not use words but acts, whose meaning is often understood only when it is too late. For example, they may give away cherished possessions, withdraw from pleasurable activities without a clear justification, or make unusual donations.

In approximately half of all suicides, the victims have consulted their GP in the months prior to death and, in an embarrassing number of cases, in the week before. It is true that many of those patients do not mention suicide to the doctors. Sometimes they report vague feeling of worthlessness or a tangential allusion to not being anymore in this world; on fewer occasions they may be quite open. It seems reasonable to think that, more than a solution to their existential problems, they are looking for empathy and human 'contact'. Needless to say, doctors should not constitute the last ring in a chain of previous disillusionments. They should not think, for example, that those who talk about suicide never do it. Nor should they abstain from raising questions about possible suicide ideation, fearing that doing so may precipitate suicidality. Research teaches that both these positions are wrong, and more professional training would be beneficial in eliminating these dangerous attitudes. Surely it is more difficult to instil the need for more attention and sensitivity, especially where heavy workloads allow only very limited time to be given to each patient (ten minutes, maybe less?). It would be rather presumptuous to think that, as doctors, we are always able to identify those patients who need more attention and more time.

It is also true that there are people who do not want to be intercepted or rescued. They want to die, perhaps to avoid endless physical suffering. There are many well-known cases of this type. Nico Speijer, an emeritus professor of psychiatry in the Netherlands and the president of the Dutch Association for Suicide Prevention, is an example. Refusing to be turned into a zombie by the medication he needed to control his pain (he suffered from cancer), he decided to die. His wife of many years committed suicide with him: they jumped together in front of a train. Sigmund Freud, in one of the most famous cases of assisted suicide, convinced his doctor, Max Schur, that he could not stand anymore the terrible suffering that the cancer at his jaw was giving him. He finally obtained a lethal dose of morphine.

Hypothetically, if we were able to stop the suffering, whatever its origin, very few people would ever contemplate suicide. Death is just the medium to avoid the continuation of the unbearable. In the case of physical suffering, palliative care is often 'too palliative' to be considered an acceptable way to live. Many patients want to retain their mental integrity, but the available protocols cannot always respect this requirement. Long-lasting, endless psychological suffering in some cases may be even more difficult to counteract. Society is much divided on these arguments, in which science is only one of the players; religious beliefs, moral values and of course laws have far more important roles.

Present-day society considers the choice of dying to be acceptable in only very few situations. For example, it can be acceptable (and even noble) to sacrifice one's own life to save the life of others, or to die for one's own country (I am afraid that 'terrorist suicide' is a common example of this). However, not all members of the community think the same way regarding these problems. Youth, for example, have a very different approach to issues. In general, they are more open to suicide, assisted suicide and euthanasia, especially if life conditions became critical due to poverty or isolation, severe physical illness, a terminal condition, and even extreme advanced age.

On the other hand, youth challenge life in many ways. Reckless and risk-taking behaviours, including extreme sports, are far more common in youngsters than in adults. The very high rate of attempted suicide in this age group is self-explanatory: the ratio of attempted to completed suicide can reach two hundred to one in youth, compared with eight to one in middle-age and two to one in the elderly.

A suicide attempt is not a form of behaviour like any other. At the very least, it is the sign of a disturbed balance. More than ten per cent of all suicide attempters eventually end their life through a fatal act, a mortality rate that today is higher than Hodgkin's lymphoma. However, these troubled people receive one-tenth of the medical attention dedicated to those who have developed Hodgkin's disease. In fact, attempters are frequently 'healthy' individuals who have deliberately provoked a condition often requiring medical consideration; consequently, they have to face some hostility once in an emergency ward. Medical staff may be busy coping with badly injured victims of road accidents, strokes, cardiac arrests, and the like, and there is little time to understand the tormented complexities of those who have endangered their lives in response to existential problems.

Roughly speaking, suicide attempters can be categorised into two broad groups: the 'manipulators' (those who tried to change their environment through the act), and the 'serious attempters' (those who survived by chance): the former represent most occurrences. Further effort would perhaps help to identify a third group in between, ambivalent and confused, unclear whether they really intended to die or simply wanted to communicate their despair. It is evident that this outcome-oriented perspective totally ignores the need for a deeper journey into the disordered world of suicide attempters.

Paradoxically, only a minority of suicide attempters receive the 'benefits' of a categorisation. First, only one-third are treated in emergency wards. There they receive attention only for their physical condition. After that, a number of them are directly discharged. Larger proportions are referred to a psychiatric unit for assessment and evaluation. What happens then is left to good intentions. In practice, very few suicide attempters receive effective treatment and monitoring. The problem is that, for them, the risk of a new attempt or a fatal repetition is increased in the first months after the initial episode. They should really receive extra attention.

Only a percentage of suicide attempters have a diagnosable psychiatric condition. In addition, most refuse the psychiatric perspective. Their life is sick, not necessarily their mind. So who should take care of them?

There are so many suicide attempters that one might have the impression of facing some sort of dissemination of the culture of death. And in fact, the more suicidal behaviour is adopted as a problem-solving strategy in crisis situations, the more this 'solution' is imitated. For example, if a mother attempts suicide in a moment of personal difficulties, the probability of a child following her example is very high — far bigger than in a family without such an experience.

Youth are particularly exposed to imitative behaviour, as the literature on the effects of media on suicidal phenomena clearly indicates. They are vulnerable individuals subject to all sorts of pressures and expectations, not yet equipped with the experience that would be necessary to properly cope with most existential difficulties. Not only do they have to deal with a changing body and the search for comfortable gender identification, but also with feelings and emotions whose deflagrating impact may turn their lives into heaven or hell in a blink. Males, in particular, are forced to be successful everywhere: at school, in sports activities, socially and financially. Always smiling, energetic and aggressive, their muscles sculpted and well identifiable under their clothes, they mustn't betray the slightest weakness or uncertainty. Isn't this too much to expect? Quite paradoxically, males have also to 'succeed' in their suicide attempt. Females can 'fail': this is accepted. But men's attempts have to result in death. It is a cultural script. A very cruel one.

Today, everybody demands the right to the best possible quality of life. This is perfectly legitimate, even if it may render us bit by bit more superficial, and — what is far worse — push all of us towards an unrestrained individualism, affecting all ages.

Parents, for example, are trying to do their best with their children, I believe. The problem is that sometimes this is not enough. Too often the focus is on lifestyle rather than children's real emotional needs. What is needed, I think, is real attention, understanding and acceptance. We do not have to share the views of our children or to approve their choices; it is more important to show that we are accepting them, with their doubts, weaknesses and mistakes. To children, their parents are the most important people in the world. From the awareness of being accepted by Mum and Dad, they develop confidence in being accepted outside the family.

Sometimes, diaries or other material brought to my attention by parents of suicide victims show that those children felt they received no consideration within the family — that they counted for nothing. They actually had received at least a 'normal' amount of nurture/attention/love from their parents, but their perception of it was too distorted. They thought that, after they suicided, their father, mother, brothers and sisters would continue their usual lives, maybe even better than before. And this added to their dissatisfaction and anger, increasing their determination to act. These children did not hate their parents and siblings; on the contrary, they loved them. But they could not see any future happiness for themselves; they felt there was no room in the world for them, and that they were not needed at all.

During the more than two decades I have dedicated to the study of suicidal behaviour, many people have offered me their personal accounts of what happened to them. Probably, they just wanted me to understand better. Some of them have even said to me, 'If you promise to read it, next time I'll bring with me the story of what I went through'. And normally I promise.

At the beginning, I was just curious. Then I realised that these scripts were incredibly important documents. They were spontaneous reports, untouched by the medical model of investigating. The stories are rather unique witnesses of tormented lives; amazing reports on what predisposed, fostered, and finally triggered the suicidal behaviour. I believe that I have now a couple of hundred of these stories in my files. Among them, there are tales of people who survived their suicide attempt just by chance. Some of these cases are excellent examples of life resurrection: wars that have finally been won, even if sometimes at a very high cost. In this perspective, they may represent a magnificent, non-traditional opportunity for understanding suicide and preventing it. But they are also evidence of the role of impulsivity, the influence of psychiatric conditions, and the terrible impact of stigma. In some of the stories, it is difficult not to interpret the suicidal choice as coldly rational.

In this book, I have selected stories representative of a variety of different situations, and of course those for which permission for reproduction exists. I often receive stories by mail and through the Internet. Only one of these is here reported, because of its peculiarity and the touching message that accompanied it. Obviously, having personal knowledge of a given subject helps a lot in understanding their individual story.

Some of the authors wanted their names clearly reported; some others preferred to remain unidentified and so a pseudonym has been used. In the selection that I have put together there are stories from both Australians and Italians. Each tale is followed by a brief comment; nothing really technical, just a way to provide the reader with a user-friendly roadmap that may assist with guidance through the many messages that the accounts convey.

The book opens with 'Sharks and Dolphins', a chapter from a professional writer, Cynthia Morton, that I have solicited after meeting her. This lady is a brilliant communicator and motivational speaker; she has already published an autobiography, and more. She certainly has the capacity to capture the reader's attention. The fresh style of her narration counterbalances the many miseries of her past life. Today

Cynthia is very active in helping people with her famous *Emotional Fitness* program.

I have never met Trevor, the author of 'A Job in the Army', but I was captivated by his terrible story, which he sent to me via the web. In my professional life I have encountered a number of situations reminiscent of Trevor's case, a person who suffered tremendous consequences from his deadly suicide attempt.

'Proxies' is the story of Anna, and describes the role of sexual abuse as an antecedent of suicidal behaviour. If perpetrators of this kind of violence were more aware of the long-term, devastating effects of their actions, perhaps the number of these crimes would be reduced.

In 'The Box of Biscuits', a beautiful young lady, Alessa, describes the series of life events that nearly destroyed her. Her case exemplifies a number of important factors that usually increase the risk of suicidal behaviour: the learning of suicide as a problem-solving strategy, the terrible impact that psychiatric conditions can produce on people, the role of negative experiences and impulsivity in conditioning life (and death), and more. This is a truly captivating story, told with a great sense of humour and irony.

'My Beautiful Grapes' is a very moving story, with unusual features, told to me by Sergio, an Italian farmer from Veneto, some years ago. I thought his story was somehow impossible. I remember that he was upset by my incredulous expression, and then he showed to me his terrible scars as proof. This man helped me to understand more about life in a rural setting and the values that are dominant in that culture.

'A Busy Husband' is the story of Lucia and underscores the role of genetics in suicide or, at least, the importance that poor control over powerful feelings may have in determining a fatal behaviour. However, there are more than biological dimensions here. Anxiety is a central player; and when this is mixed with unhappiness, dissatisfaction or depression, it can produce a very dangerous cocktail.

'The Missed Concert' is the story of Sandro, a very promising pianist with a rather peculiar character (not unusual for musicians!). As many young men do, he dealt very badly with the problem of separating from his wife. An alcohol abuser, he came close to paying a very high price for his difficulties.

A totally different tale, 'Country Living', presents Fabrizio as a man who survived 'by mistake'. His narrative, especially of the first part of his life, is interesting and moving. This story again underlines the role of issues such as inheritance, imitation, mental disorders, and negative life events in the genesis of suicidal behaviours.

In 'Afternoons on the Verandah', you may be tempted to believe, like Umberto, that 'God did not permit it'. In my files, there are similar tales, but I had to include this particular human experience. Umberto, its protagonist, died a few years ago, but from natural causes, not suicide.

I am privileged to give some permanency to the narrative from my elderly friend of 'In a Far Land'. I met her in the Geriatric Hospital of Padua, and her story still haunts me. She allowed her report to be recorded. She thought she was too old to write and not literate enough to do it properly.

Finally, contributors who survived the death of their loved ones wrote the last two stories. In 'A Familiar Smell of Garlic', Diane, the protagonist, is beset by the vision of her suicided mother. Poignantly, Diane is able to sketch the impact that the tragic death of a parent can have on the lives of surviving children.

In 'The Dream of a Life', Francesca discovered her son's body, and her tale is the description of a journey through hell, and finding her way out.

All these stories speak loudly about the possibility of a new start after existential tsunamis. They teach us that, even when everything seems lost, there still is possibility for resurrection and for finding new meanings and new ways in life.

This book is their gift to us, and the most important message of these accounts.

Diego De Leo, February, 2009

Part
TWO

❧❧

Stories from the edge

Sharks and Dolphins

Cynthia's Story

ear Diego,

Being suicidal at different phases in life does not mean we are always destined to feel that way. My story illustrates that fact.

From as far back as I can remember, I always wanted to 'get dead'. I understood at four years of age that when people 'got dead', they did not come back to earth, they left forever, and that was what I so desperately craved to do as a little girl. I wanted to go home, and the house I lived in with my biological family was not home to my heart. The sky was home.

I spent many, many hours lying on Mother Earth so that she could hold me, and nurture me, and I could feel her secret and silent energy recharge my bruised and abused little body with her gentle and loving life-force. Like a drained battery in need of recharging, her magnetic field discreetly hummed through my small body with a healing vibration that I have difficulty explaining. Mother Nature was my heart's true parent; I could always rely on her to listen, love and show me hope and beauty. Sometimes it would be through the delicious colour of a flower, the cuteness of a sparrow's tummy feathers breathing in and out. Or maybe through her loving eyes that disguised themselves, to those not in the know, as clouds and stars.

It is only now at age 40, looking back on those days, do I truly understand that I was a suicidal child, then teenager and later adult. I feel like I courted death all throughout my life. Like an elusive lover, I waited desperately for him to send me a signal, or to just show up and take me away from it all, but he never showed. I laid the red carpet out for him many times, inviting him into my life; I dreamt about him constantly, about his exquisite touch that brought relief. I longed to be with him, but I was always faced with rejection. Death represented freedom. I felt jailed, jailed in Ken and Barbie land.

My home was in an Adelaide suburb in Australia, ironically called Paradise. It was Ken and Barbie land to me and anything but a paradise. My mother was gorgeous. Physically perfect in every way, and anything that wasn't perfect about her she had changed with plastic surgery, even back in the 1960s. She was a babe — one of those women who turned men's heads wherever she went. Her fashion sense was impeccable, with her groovy zigzag patterned purple and black mini-skirts, beehive hairstyle, perfectly applied black-cat eyeliner and the knee high 'come and get me' boots accessorised with her voluptuous Sophia Loren-styled cleavage. She always had those yellow cylinder containers with red lids in her purse and in the bathroom — Ford pills, diet pills — she ate them like lollies. She was always a very busy lady, with not much time to spare and lots to do. She was a hairdresser from home and had a constant flow of women in and out of our house that demanded her full attention.

My dad, well, he was the rugged GI Joe-style Ken doll. He had craggy Charles Bronson-like features, dark hair, olive skin; a thickset, charismatic, but angry man. He was a ladies man, a charmer — and his name really was Ken, so I didn't stand a chance; it really was Ken and Barbie land. We looked like perfection on the exterior, with me and my older sister always immaculately dressed, with our hair curled and styled, with colour coordinated bows to match our dresses, frilly white socks and shiny black patent Mary-Jane style shoes. We looked flawless whenever the family ventured out. However, the interior world of the household was very different, riddled with violence, alcoholism, loud yelling and incest, blended with a great deal of pretence and denial — we were all good at keeping up appearances.

It was not only my incestuous relationship with my father that made suicide seem like an attractive option, nor the violence that was conveniently called discipline or 'tough love,' but also the paedophile who baby-sat me on a regular basis. He lived next door to us in Paradise. He really was the icing on the cake, and made all human beings inside and outside my house seem unsafe or untouchable. Living was unattractive to me. I did not like humans at all. They all seemed like emotional sharks.

Safe or unsafe?

I use the terms 'emotional sharks' and 'emotional dolphins' regularly today with my writing and public-speaking career. I initially created these titles after looking into the eyes of abused children I work with and for whom I am proudly an Ambassador. These kids cared for by the Kids First Foundation are aged from three to five years, and have lived in emotional war zones with sharks like I did as a child. As far as they are concerned, the world is full of only sharks — unsafe people who harm. They need to believe that emotional dolphins also exist — safe people who can help them. However, in learning how to tell the difference between the two one cannot go by visual appearances, or by looks. Emotional sharks and emotional dolphins both look the same. All the kids called the very sick paedophile that lived next door Uncle Roy; he was a safe-looking man. He was a silver-haired chap in his fifties who was friendly, clean and very neighbourly. He was a married man who lived with his wife and had grown children. He would take neighbours' garbage out without being asked, mow your lawn for you when you were away on holidays, collect the mail, and oh yes, of course, mind your children for you anytime — gladly.

As a little girl, I was always told about stranger danger, or those bad men, and to stay away from them. Bad people, or sharks, were the men in the park who were dirty and unshaven in an old smelly raincoat and wanted to give you lollies. I was warned about these dangerous individuals, but not about Daddy or Uncle Roy. So you see it is deceptive to rely on looks alone to tell a shark from a dolphin, as they both have grey fins. You have to be able to rely on how people make you feel, safe or unsafe. And if a child lives in a home where no adult is emotionally available, because they are always too busy or drinking and/or drugging, feelings are an inconvenience or they are unable to be felt. So if a child's feelings are ignored and not validated, the child learns to ignore nature's intuition and dismiss feelings as being useful alarms. The only choice is to then measure life by the material or physical, how something looks or what it is worth. That is what I learned.

This is not about blaming my parents, because parents cannot pass on information to their children they do not have, and if grandparents are emotionally unavailable so too will be the parents and the children, until someone breaks the cycle. Parents are still only now, 40 years on from my abuse, becoming educated about this silent problem. I was astounded when I first started writing and working in this field to discover the appalling statistics that are readily available elsewhere.

Not liking humans as a little girl was my reality — they confused me, hurt me and I felt bad, wrong, silly and dirty around them. I didn't like being one of them myself. I wanted to fly away like my friends the sparrows, to my home in the sky beyond the clouds and stars, into the eyes of Mother Nature.

Being suicidal at age four, my attempts were never successful but, by God, I kept trying — I did not give up. One of my naive techniques was eating the red sulphur off the top of matches. It occurred to me while watching my father pick his teeth with a match he had whittled down into a toothpick, and I decided to imitate him. My grandmother spotted me with the red sulphur end of a match in my mouth and sharply told me that young ladies did not pick their teeth and that the red end of the match was poisonous and dangerous and never to put it in my mouth. Well, in my four-year-old worldliness I had learned that 'poisonous' and 'dangerous' could 'get you dead' and that was my aim. From that day onward I stole boxes of matches whenever I could — and in a house with a father as a smoker it was easy pickings. I would hide them with my dolls clothes and then secretly eat them, devouring each one with delight and excitement. I would then go out and lie on the grass and wait to 'get dead' and to be taken up into the sky, away from this horrible place called my home. But obviously it did not happen. I would get an upset stomach but did not 'get dead'. I also tried running into traffic on the way to school, and during morning recess I would leave school and run home. I would run across busy main roads with no fear, hoping to get hit and get off the planet, but cars screeched to a stop, I got yelled at and my parents got phoned from the school ... but I never got dead!

My dad was a shark most of the time throughout my childhood and brought much insanity, pain and confusion to my life, but those moments when he was in dolphin mode — for me as his daughter were truly divine. He was my favourite person on the planet. He was a wonderful wordsmith — a talented poet and writer and a wonderful cartoonist, a true natural. I understood his pain. He, too, was abused in childhood. I know this because when he abused me, he would talk to the voices in his head that had abused him; he would use my little body in some twisted way to get revenge on them.

Then he would put his head next to mine on my pillow and sob and say sorry to me and tell me that he loved me, and sometimes he would even thank me. I felt very important to him, very special, his true love at four years of age. My mother and sister were the enemy, for they did not know him like I did; he loved me the most, he told me, and it was our secret. I would never tell; they would be too sad, he told me, and I did not want to be mean, they would not understand. But I hated him too. I hated the way he would disregard me the next morning and pretend like nothing had happened. He would hit me and tell me I was a scatterbrain, I disgusted him and he let me know it. I was in a constant state of confusion.

A great start?

Much of my teenage years is a blur. My parent's violence and drinking escalated and so did my father's infidelities. We left Adelaide and moved to Brisbane to start a fresh, but my father's habits did not change. I was aged thirteen when we moved interstate. My sexual abuse stopped with Uncle Roy at age seven (when we moved house) and ceased with my father at age nine. It was just after this that my baby brother was born, eight years my junior. I now understand that paedophiles need young bodies to arouse them and mine was obviously getting too big. I was very concerned for my baby brother's sexual and physical safety and so became his inseparable personal guard. We were almost joined at the hip, and even though he was younger, I found enjoyment and safety for the first time ever in his humanity. He was a wonderful breath of fresh air in my toxic life. I was very protective of him, obsessively so.

When my father finally left the family home in Brisbane in my early teenage years, I was relieved but also devastated, as my loyalty to him ran deep. Initially, I stayed with my mother, sister and brother. It was then that I started to really utilise a delightful orange plastic typewriter I had been given a few years before. I loved that typewriter. I loved the clicking sound its case made when I opened it — it had an exciting importance about it for me. I tapped away, writing scripts for the neighbourhood children to perform on the front lawn on Sunday afternoons for all the parents to watch. I started to really get into my drawing. With portraits I was always good at the eyes. I had studied eyes all my life, learning how to read their silent language for my own survival. I could draw them really well and got a great deal of enjoyment from being good at something. It was as though my creativity could be released because I did not have to spend so much time being hyper vigilant, watching for my brother's or my own safety. The home environment was not such an unpredictable violent war zone for a while; it was great, like a holiday. Until my mother's new boyfriend came on the scene. His sexual energy was repulsive. I moved out to my father's place — better the devil you know.

My ability to recount the next few years in perfect sequence is poor. Not only I was suicidal, but drinking heavily and living with chronic, undiagnosed post-traumatic stress disorder (PTSD). Inevitably, I was very disoriented. I chose homelessness for periods of time, when living with either my mother or father became totally unmanageable for my sanity. My father's young girlfriends and his raging temper seemed harder to handle away from my mother, sister and brother; it was almost like he had open slather to be as violent as he chose. My mother's boyfriend used to try to set me up with his friends for dates; they drank heaps, and the energy was revolting. Homelessness was the best option. At one point, I hitchhiked back to Adelaide to try to make sense of my chaotic life. I also hoped that if I moved geographically I would move away from the sewer in my life, but I just took it with me, my own self-hatred and childhood trauma.

My first sexual experience with a male around my own age when I was sixteen contributed to my becoming suicidal once more. I had not really understood that I had been sexually abused as a young child. I had managed to bury most of my traumatic childhood memories in the dark caves of my heart. Having lost my physical virginity as a child without really comprehending what was happening now made sense. The male was a golden-haired surfer from the Gold Coast in Queensland. I was only attracted to blonde males who were tall and athletic. I think somewhere in my subconscious I believed that if they were physically the opposite of my father, they would be opposite in every way and never hurt me. Believing that dolphins looked different from sharks started way back then.

Of course, the blonde surfer was only interested in the sexual conquest and, as soon as it was over, he lost interest and moved onto the next girl. I cried all the way through the ordeal and was disassociated for days afterward. I did not understand what disassociation was back then. It is like being in shock, disoriented, teary and unable to communicate what is wrong — like being stoned but without feeling good, just numb and disconnected from everyone and everything. Everything that had happened with Uncle Roy and Dad came flooding back. I understood that it was not normal and is not supposed to happen between children and adults. It did not make sense ... it was my fault. I was terrified at the reality of my own life. Out of loyalty to my father whom I had promised to never tell, and genuine love for him coupled with a very real fear of his violent temper, I knew to keep my mouth shut. I did not want to stay on this planet if sex was a part of being a grown woman — I hated it — it made me feel dirty and ugly and afraid. I wanted to die once more.

My mother knew I was distressed but of course I could not tell her why; I was so angry at the world, so she took me to a local doctor. I could not tell him what was wrong with me. I was just angry and he being a male did not help. I think I was demanding and rude to him. He prescribed sedatives and told me I needed to calm down. I demanded to see someone else immediately, someone who could really help me. He replied that a tantrum would do me no good with him, that people do not always get what they want when they want it, and that I would have to make an appointment to see someone else.

I took the whole bottle of sedatives to the public toilets. I stood at the basin staring into my own pupils for quite a while. My older sister was convinced my problem was that I was possessed by the devil. She used religion like I used alcohol; she had even taken me to a church counsellor under the pretext of helping me. It was an exorcism where I was locked in a small room with a lunatic priest chanting in Latin. As I looked at my own desperate eyes in the mirror, I wondered if I was the devil or insane or just plain stupid; maybe I was all three. I swallowed the lot, looking at myself dead in the eye, not afraid but almost trying to console myself that soon it would all be over, we could go home to Mother Nature in the sky. I calmly went into the toilet cubicle and locked the door. I lay in a foetal position around the base of the toilet and felt comforted by the cool green and white tiles beneath me. I closed my eyes and waited for death, my lover to come for me — he did not show yet again.

I awoke in an intensive care unit, very angry that I was still on the planet. I was so pissed off that I was too dumb to even kill myself. I recall sitting in a small room with my parents and a doctor. The doctor was speaking to my parents about the severity of my depression. My father sat in silence. A few short months afterward, he left Australia to live in Papua New Guinea and never returned. He died overseas when I was aged 26 and pregnant with my second son. His girlfriend, who sat in a daze on his bed as he dropped dead from a cerebral haemorrhage, was also aged 26.

I had been told all my life that I was a silly-billy, a scatter-brain — I now understand I spent much of my childhood dis-associated, and I am also dyslexic. So this dumb scatterbrain was left high and dry by death once more. My solution was to intentionally emotionally medicate more with alcohol, food, and, in my thirties, drugs.

Reinventing the wheel

I only found out the dyslexia at 39 years of age. I just always thought I was dumb because I can write about my inner world — no problems — but with anything else, like an exam paper or proposal, I am lost. I thought dyslexic people could not write at all nor read. I now understand through my psychiatrist that dyslexia manifests in many different forms. I am unable to retain the written word, to read and comprehend what I have read. I am able to parrot words back, but have no retentive ability whatsoever of the written word.

It is like a scrambler goes on whenever I read and the words fall through the holes in my brain. That is why I do so poorly in any left-brain activity. All throughout school I would get perhaps 2 out of 100 questions correct in Maths, and that was just plain lucky guessing. I can hold words for a little while with a coloured highlighter pen; any book I attempt to read ends up tattooed with colour on the point I attempt to retain. However, when I write it is like a dam breaks and words just flow so easily. When people who had purchased my first book asked me about what I had written in the second chapter, or quoted a page number, I had absolutely no recall about what I had written.

I met a Ken doll of my own and married him in my early twenties. We had two sons within 21 months of each other and I became drunk on motherhood — a true smother mother. I abstained from heavy drinking throughout my pregnancies and their early years. They were some of the best years of my life ... but I used food. My weight at five foot ten inches has fluctuated from 59 kilos to 97 kilos. Like a true addict, if I put one addiction down another pops up its ugly head to be dealt with. Anything that hits a pleasure centre in my brain I have to be very careful about. Drugs, alcohol, sex, food, money — I can use any or all of them to destroy my life. My capacity to say enough or moderate is impaired, so I have to learn that some substances I have to totally abstain from and others I need to monitor carefully.

By the time my two sons were aged seven and nine and both at school, I got back into heavy drinking of alcohol, but added drugs. I did not know how to fill up my days without the boys being at home, and my drinking was getting out of hand by this stage. I was becoming violent, having bad blackouts and not getting much relief. I noticed that people who used drugs tended to drink less and be quieter; I thought I would give it a go.

I had recreated the perfect Ken and Barbie world once more, and I myself attempted to be the best Barbie I knew how. Pamela Anderson became the ultimate role model for me. She was the perfect sexualised Barbie doll symbol to me then. I attempted to become like her. Big blonde hair, breast implants, fake tan, false fingernails, baby doll clothes, and a steady diet of drugs, alcohol, diet pills, caffeine and cigarettes, with as little food as possible.

The Barbie doll mother who picked up her sons from school in those days was indeed a sad picture. I would stagger out of the car after roaring into the school car park with music blaring so loud the car doors would vibrate. Stumbling on my high heels over the gravel in the car park, I would attempt to sashay up to my sons' class rooms to meet them, finding walking a straight line almost impossible. I had been to lunch with the girls, drinking and drugging. My mini-skirt was tucked into my undies, my cleavage falling out of my baby doll pink top, my hair wild, focus blurred, winking at the teacher. My poor babies, I'm sure, would cringe to themselves and think, 'My God here comes our mother'. A woman with huge cleavage, a short mini-skirt, flirting with the men, living on diet pills, needing alcohol to socialise and relying on plastic surgery to give her more self-esteem. I had become my mother.

The wise old gum tree

My last night of using drugs was on October 11, 1995. I had Ken and Barbie land perfect at this stage. The house was tidy, the children were well-dressed and I weighed in at the lowest weight I had ever managed to reach, 59 kilos. I had four kilos to go to be really perfect though. Elle McPherson was a few inches taller than me; I had read in one of my gossip-bible tabloid magazines that she only weighed 55 kilos. So I needed to up my diet pills; I had some serious starving to do.

We were at a dinner party surrounded by professional people, pilots and doctors, all flirting with each other's wives and husbands. We were drinking great duty-free booze and doing some nice drugs. However, I had started at midday to get a run-up to be able to cope with a social engagement. By 11 pm that evening, after almost 12 hours of solid using, I was still not drunk or high. It was then my suicide plug came out once more. It literally felt like a plug in the gut of my stomach had come out and emotional sewerage began filling me up from the inside. I felt it rise up through my chest making my heart pound with panic, as if it were about to drown me at any moment. The heavy lump in my throat grew, and I could almost gag with the repulsive taste of my own reality. My eyes became heavy and I so desperately wanted to cut myself — to cut my skin and let all the sewerage that was poisoning me out so I could have some relief.

I wanted to get out of my own skin — escape the jail that was me. I looked around the table at these strangers laughing and talking and I could not hear them — I knew they did not see me — I did not know me nor did I want to, for I was just a sewer, a wreck. Once more I wanted my lover Death to come and rescue me from this bad joke called my life. I vaguely recall pulling my husband into the toilet to have sex with me to try to distract myself from my despair. He obliged but I felt sadder somehow afterward. Sex was a form of validation that I had worth, and I used it from time to time to help my self-esteem. Usually, I felt like at least I was good at something afterwards, but not this time. I also used sex to feed my desperate pretence that my marriage was okay. I measured my value as a wife and the quality of our marriage by the amount of sex we had. I had to believe that the marriage that had the most sex was the best sort. I so desperately wanted to be the best at something.

In those days I did not fall asleep or wake up, I passed out and came to. That night I don't recall where or how I passed out. But I came to the next morning in my bed at around 10 a.m. The house was silent — the boys had been taken to school, it was a Friday morning. I opened my puffy eyes to see drugs and alcohol next to the bed and an overflowing ashtray. My hair was matted with vomit and leaves; I was naked but could not remember where my clothes were. I was bruised and stiff as though I had fallen down a flight of stairs, but had no recollection of why I felt so battered. My eyes were almost purple with broken blood vessels around them from the forced violent vomiting I knew I demanded of myself, often if I had eaten a meal during my drinking and drugging sessions. If I stood, alcoholic diarrhoea would involuntarily run down my legs — I was 33 years of age and a shipwreck of a human being.

There was a wise old gum tree that stood tall and proud outside my bedroom window. It was one of those gums whose bark is smooth to touch and almost white. It had a beautiful long arm that seemed to be outstretched as if attempting to cradle the bedroom section of our house. It was also the home of a wonderful owl that used to come and visit me from time to time — I chose to believe it was there to watch over me and silently remind me that Mother Nature was calling me to come home to her. Then I thought that meant suicide; now I know she was beckoning me to come home to my own heart.

That morning the owl was not there, but that beautiful outstretched arm seemed to be magnetically pulling me to come and rest my weary head on the breast of its trunk. As I cradled my knees, naked, bruised and mute on my bed that morning, suicidal thoughts seduced me relentlessly.

During the past week leading up to this morning, I had been fantasising once more about Death — my absent lover — and our hopefully forthcoming rendezvous. The problem was I was not going to be able to run away with him without my two boys. I was spiritually unable to leave my babies. During that last week of my drinking and drugging I was not getting any relief from anything, so suicide (that tantalising affair) was becoming my only avenue of escape. I actually picked a location where I could drive my car off the freeway into the Brisbane River. I felt relief as I pictured in my mind's eye the water level rising up the car windows as we sank and knowing that we were all going home to Mother Nature — to a better place beyond the clouds and stars. My boys were going to be with me and I thought in all my insanity that it was the most responsible action, to take them with me, for the world was full of sharks and no one could protect them except me. I don't feel wonderful as I type these words, but that honestly was my level of sanity on October 12, 1995; but I did not agree to do a chapter in this book to be liked, but to be useful. I had run out of hope and could feel no love, nor see any beauty, or reason to stay on the planet. My sons' seven- and nine-year-old faces kept coming to mind as I contemplated the choice of life or death once more. I could not speak. Hot, heavy tears that felt like blood ran down my cheeks, I was so very, very lost. I looked up at that beautiful outstretched arm and I spoke to her — to Mother Nature, my heart's parent. I did not speak to her as a companion as I always had when we silently chatted in the past, but this time

I asked her to help me. I had never felt worthy of ever asking her for a favour and I wasn't asking for myself, I was asking for my babies, my beautiful sons who deserved a chance at a life with a dolphin mother. They deserved a chance far more than I believed I did.

I spoke out loud to the tree on that morning asking for help. That was just over seven years ago when I typed these words in November 2002. I have not picked up a drink or a drug from that day to this but much has changed — I dumped Death, that unreliable lover, I now have a love affair with Life. However it has not been a bed of roses; I had to put manure on my heart's garden bed first before the roses bloomed. It was not pretty for a while, and it seemed that roses would never bud — but they did in time.

Six weeks into my recovery I began to feel the seeds of self-respect take root. The boys would get into the car and be wide-eyed with smiles as they noticed their mother had not been kidnapped by drugs and alcohol again and that I was emotionally available to be with them and ask them about their day. I began to notice freckles on their noses I had never seen before and understood for the first time that these boys had seen way too much violence and irresponsible addictive behaviour in their short lives. Self-respect was a totally new feeling for me and I did not want to lose it. I needed to break the cycle, for my children had been living in the same environment that I have had as a child and they deserved so much more.

My marriage, however, did not function without drugs and alcohol. The man I was married to felt like an absolute stranger. I did not know how to talk to him — I felt too embarrassed to get changed in front of him and sex with him was too difficult and confronting to even contemplate. Our marriage ended when I was six weeks clean and sober. I was unable to continue being the party girl and our lifestyle had been full of consistent social engagements — our home had been nicknamed 'party central'.

Dolphin people

I became a single mother and lived on a pension with my two boys in a quarter of a rented house near their school. I had met my first dolphin woman, Barbara, when I was just ten days clean and sober. She became my heart's lifeline and my mentor. Dolphin people, being safe people, don't just say things — they live them.

She showed me that love is an action not a word, it is what you do, not what you say that counts. My social circle disappeared, and I needed to remove myself from my biological family to stay sane. My mother's new verbally abusive alcoholic boyfriend was not one whom I wanted my children around and her daily drinking made it hard for me to be around her. Barbara brought me a new doona for my bed when I moved away from my husband, because the old one still had his scent on it; I cried myself to sleep every night. She bought me a beautiful fragrance to wear every day, even though I was on the pension; it made me feel beautiful when I wore it, I got pleasure the whole day through from the gentle floral scent. She would speak to me lovingly at 2 a.m. when I was distraught with childhood memory, a true dolphin. She did more for me than I can ever put into words and still continues to do so today. She has become my mother figure and my boy's grandmother figure, she models grace, and integrity, and dignity and I hope to grow more like her in the years to come.

At 16 months clean and sober I was put into a psychiatric hospital. I had chronic PTSD but did not know it; I just thought I was going slowly crazy. The symptoms began happening regularly and kept escalating. I could be standing in a supermarket cue waiting to pay for my groceries and the man standing next to me may have had the same nasal hair as Uncle Roy. A tidal wave of trauma would hit me. I would lose my capacity to speak or stand. I would fall to the floor in a foetal position no matter where I was. I became mute, I could not speak, I began hyperventilating, my eyes would be open but I could not see, it was terrifying. Then my head would play the story of the abuse in every detail, I would relive the event. It was so intense I felt like I was going to die there and then or that something inside my brain would snap and I would be insane forever.

Thankfully my boys knew how to help. I believe the world is consistently replenished with dolphin love in the form of children and animals every day. A child or an animal learns how to be an unsafe person — a shark — it is not innate. My boys' dolphin love got me to safety every time. They would pat me as if I was a distressed puppy and tell me in their most reassuring voices that they would not leave me, nor let anyone get me, that I was safe and they were calling Barbara and that she would come and help us. Barbara always came.

Eventually, the PTSD got so chronic that I was put into a psychiatric hospital. I was 16 months clean and sober and had left my using environment, the violence, and all the sharks in my life. I had been working on a Twelve-Step program with my sponsor Barbara and now I was in a loony bin. I did not get it! Now in hindsight I understand that Twelve-Step programs are brilliant for drug and alcohol problems, but they are not designed to heal abuse, cancer, Aids, depression or mental ill-nesses. I needed more help, and help was the hardest thing for me to ask for.

It was in this hospital, wedged between the wardrobe and the wall, sitting on the ground holding my knees, wearing my stylish hospital gown with the bows at the back, when the shark in my own head was at its worst. It was telling me that I was going to lose custody of my boys and that I was too stupid to kill myself, so I would probably spend the rest of my days a dribbling crazy woman in a psych ward. I had finally understood that my suicide attempts to be with my elusive lover Death were just a waste of time. But living a normal life seemed just as hopeless too.

My beautiful Barbara had brought me in some beautiful yellow roses and placed them next to my hospital bed. She also brought in photos of my boys and of Glenn, a beautiful dolphin man who had entered my life and was attempting to love me. The beauty of their faces and those roses eventually overrode the shark's dialogue in my head. I began to recall how I used colour and flowers as a child to calm myself when life was too hard. Beauty had been a sanity saver then, and it was working again now. I believe that human beings are wired to love beauty. So if I could see beauty I would feel feelings of love, for that beauty and love leads to hope, the hope that maybe more beauty is available to be enjoyed another day. If there is love, even if it is for a flower or a child, it can be a reason to go on, to want to live for just one more day. Well, that is how it was for me.

Chatting to the roses

I eventually got out from in-between the wardrobe and the wall and had a chat to the roses. I still speak to flowers and trees and the sky today, sometimes out loud, and sometimes just with my heart in a secret silent language. I asked Mother Nature for a deal this time. I asked her to help me not lose custody of my boys and to get me out of there, and I promised to spend the rest of my life helping people understand about the plight of the addicted and the abused. The next day I was introduced to yet another shrink, but this one was different. A dolphin. He told me I was not crazy and did not belong in that hospital. He explained I had chronic PTSD and if I gave him five to seven years we could work through it. He said we were going to start my treatment without medication and see how we went. He was a father himself and in love with his wife; I could see it in his eyes. My hope grew.

I began to write while living with Glenn, and to paint and see my shrink every week. I also began to work voluntarily on a help line. I eventually took my rough notes to my doctor while having a check-up and she read through them. She said that she would endorse my work, for she believed that many of her clients and colleagues would benefit from my writing. She was the president of the Australian Medical Association at the time in Queensland; I was thrilled to have her validation.

I got a loan on a credit card and went to a photocopy place and ran off as many copies as we could afford. We spent over $5000 in the process. I then distributed the books and approached a large chain of bookstores in Brisbane. They liked the book, calling it a 'boutique style of book' and put it in ten of their stores. By the second week it was in store, it hit the top 10 bestseller list, at number 8. The third week it was in store it climbed to number 4, heading I hoped for number one. The next week the chain of bookstores went bankrupt and had to close their doors. Much of the money from my book sales would take quite some time if it was ever going to get to me; I owed the printers $5000 and could not pay. Of course, the shark in my head was telling me that only bad things will happen to me if I try to belong, because I don't, I am a bad and stupid person. Well, I had just written a book on how to listen to the dolphin and override the shark so I took some of my own advice and followed my heart and listened to the dolphins around me who urged me to continue.

I decided to try a real publishing house. I knew the deal — I was unpublished, unknown and I did not have an agent. Addiction and abuse were also difficult subjects to encourage people to read about. I felt I would be lucky if I even got to speak to the editor's secretary, and my book would probably be placed in a six-month long queue to maybe be considered. But nonetheless it was worth a try. I also knew my grammar may be an issue, and even though my 13-year-old son had done the editing for me, it was still pretty rough.

I will never forget the two weeks my son took to edit my work. He had been the dux of his school and was excellent at English. The book sat on his bedside table seemingly untouched. I was unsure if he really wanted to do it for me even though he had offered. Reading about his mother's journey could well have been way too confronting a task for him. The weeks continued to pass until one day he walked into the laundry as I was separating the clothes for washing. He stood at the laundry door with the book pressed to his chest and quietly said: 'Mum, I've read and edited your book for you'. My heart was pounding and I was hoping that, he was okay. He then went on to say: 'Mum, I've done your corrections with red pen, there are quite a few'. And then he paused: 'One more thing Mum I just have to say, after having read your book', he then looked me dead in the eye and said: 'Mum, I really like you'. I will never forget those words and knew from that moment on that no matter what came out of this book, my son knew his mother's warts and all and still liked her regardless.

So I made the phone call and hoped to be put through to the editor's secretary. I was surprised when I was put through without too much interrogation. The phone rang a couple of times and then a woman with a very polished English accent answered. I introduced myself and blabbed on about my little book and it making the top 10 bestseller list in Brisbane in its photocopied format. When I had finished, she then explained that she was not the editor's secretary but in fact the editor. Her secretary was in the ladies room, and she commented that she rarely answered her phone for her, but just decided to do so on this occasion. She asked me to pop my book in the mail and let her have a look at it. I was gobsmacked. On receiving my book, she then sent me air tickets and cab vouchers to come to Sydney to meet her. She said she would not publish anyone she did not like, so she needed to meet with me face-to-face.

We met; she offered me a publishing contract and my book hit bookstores nationally. I began doing a great deal of publicity including radio and magazine interviews and television guest appearances. My public-speaking career then took off, as did my artwork. I was astounded when an art gallery owner saw my work and wanted to include it in an exhibition. I explained to her that it was emotional vomiting, and she explained to me that was what art was. I had no idea. These days my work is auctioned for children's charities, and I am invited to exhibit my work for all sorts of worthwhile events.

I married that beautiful dolphin man, Glenn; we have been married for five years now. My boys hog the camera when media come to our home, a far cry from the days when they cringed at the sight of their mother picking them up from school. These days they want the world to know that their mother helps other kids get their mothers back.

The key points

When you invited me to contribute a chapter to this book, Diego, you asked me what were the key points, the events that lead up to me changing paths, from seeking death to seeking life. There have been many different contributing factors but they are all related to my senses — sight, smell, taste, touch and sound. My senses keep me anchored and help me to make sense of my life and know my truth. They also help me sort out the sharks from the dolphins.

As a child, my senses were useless. I could not use them to keep myself safe, they were dismissed by the adults around me. When I started to drink and then use drugs, my senses were completely numb. I could not feel or see anything, and I loved it that way for quite a long time. Drugs and alcohol were my solution for a long time before they became my problem.

When I got into recovery I needed to learn how to reconnect to myself, to learn about me, for I was a complete stranger. I did not understand that my childhood issues were not me. I did not know I could separate myself from them. I like to use the analogy of a stereo that plays a CD over and over that I hated. This music played day and night relentlessly — this horrible music represents my trauma. I was desperate to find earplugs, and drugs and alcohol worked for a while. The problem was the music kept getting louder and I could hear it through the earplugs. I had not been taught that I am not the CD, but the stereo. I did not understand they were separate items; that my abuse was a separate item to my soul, to who I was as a human being. For many years, it defined me: suicide was for me about throwing the whole stereo unit out of the window and smashing it to stop the music; to give me relief, and if that meant killing myself I was prepared to do that, anything for relief. I now understand that the stereo has a stop and an eject button and anytime the shark in my head puts on a CD that I dislike, I have a choice: I can eject it and put on some music I love and enjoy.

My senses are that tool. Pleasant sights, sounds, touch, tastes and smells actually stop the shark CD playing. I have spent the past years using colours I love, playing music I love to hear, putting photos of people I love on refrigerator doors, next to my computer, my bed, in my wallet anywhere where they can serve as validation that I am loved — which is the opposite to what my shark tries to convince me of. I put words I love to read up around the place also. I take walks, lie on Mother Earth, keep safe food around me and have loved planting my own vegetable and herb gardens.

I learned 'safe touch' for the first time through my baby brother, then my boys, then Barbara and now Glenn. I also have a masseuse whom I try to see regularly, for safe therapeutic touch is an important part of my recovery. I paint whenever I can and draw and release my creative energy. I write every single day at the close of my day; I unload any shark energy I have with words or colour and do not let it build up or play that CD for a second longer than necessary.

The most important ingredient in my recovery has been dolphin love. And the dolphins in my life have loved me and believed in me until I could love and believe in myself. I blame no one for the self-abuse I brought on to myself. I was most definitely the most destructive shark in my own life. I carried self-abuse on in my own life for decades after it actually stopped. Sharks and dolphins have both been important in my life. I am in no danger of becoming a saint or a dolphin every waking moment of my life. But I have learned how I can increase dolphin love toward myself and eject the shark's relentless tormenting CD without having to throw myself — the stereo — out the window. Sex no longer makes me feel dirty, ugly or afraid. I can now make love and smile at my darling husband in the process. I feel beautiful, loved and peaceful afterwards.

Miracles happen every day, Diego, and I am grateful to know I am just one of many people who do recover and reclaim their right to an abundant life.

But for those who do pass over and succeed in their suicide attempts I feel much compassion. Those who succeed are usually in so much pain that life is unbearable to live for one more minute. These are often people who have survived horrific emotional crises and very often in silence. If a human being eventually dies after having survived a horrific physical crisis such as a car accident, and living just means constant pain and they eventually die, we see it as a blessing, for they are no longer suffering. I see those who successfully suicide as experiencing a similar blessing for they are no longer in unbearable emotional pain, an invisible pain that no one but the sufferer can ever truly understand.

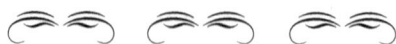

DIEGO'S COMMENTS ON CYNTHIA'S STORY

Written by the professional pen of Cynthia Morton, this beautiful tale is both powerful and captivating, and carries many important implications.

Throughout her life, Cynthia's emotions are always very powerful, and from the age of four she is conscious that she wants to 'get dead'. The red sulphur end of matches is the first possible means to exit from a life that to those outside appears 'faultless', but which is violent and threatening inside family walls.

Incest and sexual abuse from her Dad and Uncle Roy indelibly mark Cynthia's young life, and create the grounds for her division of human beings into sharks or dolphins. Her self-esteem is undermined from the very beginning, forcing her into a puppet role in a Ken and Barbie world. Fortunately she is able to obtain some comfort and nurture from 'Mother Nature'.

Barely afloat in waters where sharks and dolphins 'look the same', and safety and loyalty are never in available, Cynthia discovers she has turned into a 'babe' just like her mother — not an image she likes to have of herself. However, she gets married, has two children and — through the permanent anaesthesia of drugs and alcohol — lives in a marriage whose quality is determined by the amount of sex involved, and where making love is a sort of self-validation procedure.

But real love is not there. At the heart of 'party central', life can be very miserable.

Self-destructive behaviour continues. Cynthia lucidly describes what is behind the 'urge' to self-cut, a form of self-harming which has become very common in the past few years, especially among young girls. When you have 'a repulsive taste' of your own reality, opening your skin and letting out all the sewerage that is 'poisoning you' gives some relief.

Despite now being a wife and a mother, Cynthia still has suicidal thoughts. However, she recognises that the presence of her two children represents an additional impediment (we like to call it 'a protective factor'). As depressed and suicidal mothers tragically do sometimes, she had fantasies of drowning herself and the two kids in the Brisbane River. In her disordered view of reality, she thinks that this would be 'the most responsible action ... [because] the world [is] full of sharks and no one could protect them except me'.

Tragically, this reasoning is quite common in cases of suicide-filicide, and I have encountered it many times in my professional life. As described by Cynthia, mothers who make this type of plan do not want their children to survive them; they think they should save them from further suffering in a bad and hostile world.

Sometimes dynamics can be more complex; I have seen cases where children were perceived as 'obstacles' by their suicidal mothers. In such situations, mothers can behave aggressively towards their child. I particularly remember the wife of a young colleague of mine who was beating her five-year-old son for no reason. Her bad behaviour soon degenerated to injuring the young boy with scissors. On investigation it was found that this usually exemplary woman, this (usually) very caring mother, was planning to jump from the top of the high-rise building where they lived. She was suffering from a psychotic episode, apparently preceded by a lengthy period of depression, which she had disguised both at work and with her husband (the latter maybe a little too involved with his cardiology). With appropriate medication she recovered promptly, but the most challenging aspect of her therapy was the re-establishment of a positive relationship with her son.

However, Cynthia bravely overcomes the suicidal crisis. With the help of 'dolphin' Barbara, she is able to survive the difficult aftermath of a marriage 'that did not function without drugs and alcohol'. However, Cynthia's struggle with her ghosts is not yet over: her recovered life is subject to panic attacks, eating disorders and chronic PTSD, which she has to overcome over the course of several years.

Meeting a good doctor, and the 'dolphin' Glenn, definitely helped Cynthia to re-anchor herself. Her new self-esteem and the discovery of fresh meaning in life is a product of the many talents and emotional robustness that Cynthia naturally possesses. Her life experiences are too important to waste: they have such potential to assist — even save — many other people. Her 'Emotional Fitness' program could not have a more credible basis. Bravo Cynthia!

THREE

A Job in the Army

Trevor's Story

ear Diego,

I have chosen to share my story with you and, through you, perhaps others for whom my story may resonate. It is been hard to write about my experience. But things are best told and not hidden away.

My name is Trevor Stewart. I am now 36 years old. I have a fiancée, three step-children and a daughter of my own aged nine months. On the 26th of June 1990 I placed a loaded shotgun underneath my chin and pulled the trigger. Somehow, I survived. Why? That is the question most asked of me for so many years now. The answer licked away deep inside me for the same number of years.

I had a very happy childhood. Often referred to as the class joker at school, I enjoyed life and got great satisfaction from making others laugh, and most times trying to turn a bad situation into one where you could have a laugh. My high school principal wrote in a reference that I was a very jovial person. I never lost that sense of humour, nor was I ever going to. I left school after completing Year 10. I had only one thing in mind and that was to join the army and retire after 20 years.

I was 18 when I joined the Army. It was the start of my dream, the start of my career. I learnt many things in the Army. In fact, I could say that I grew up in the Army. It was then when I learned to drink and take drugs that my dream started to become just that, a dream. Or rather, what it became was a nightmare. Within two years I had crashed a car at a speed of 180 kph, drunk, received two charges of drink-driving and numerous charges all related to alcohol. The Army was trying to kick me out and the police were trying to lock me up. In an attempt to save my career, I admitted myself to an Army hospital in Sydney to try to get off the grog.

After a week or so I had had enough. I was being labelled an alcoholic and I didn't like it. I wasn't an alcoholic. After all I wasn't lying in a gutter drinking from a paper bag. I wasn't drinking from dawn to dusk every day of the week. Looking back now, I was, indeed, an alcoholic. I was probably one of the worst kinds. The binge drinker who couldn't say when enough was enough. So too with the drugs. The army taught me how to be a drug user.

In 1983, drugs were rife in the Army. It was so readily available. You weren't cool if you didn't smoke dope or take LSD. It was my own choice to give the 'hard' stuff a miss. I tried it but didn't like it. It was scary not being in control of my own mind, and on many occasions it reduced me to tears. But for some reason I kept going back to it. It was then that I changed my way of thinking. I still wanted my career in the Army. I still wanted to fulfil my dream. I fought to stay in the Army and I did. The Army decided to give me a second chance, but decided that it would be best to be well away from Sydney. I got posted to Melbourne and started again. It was by chance that I was placed on a promotion course by mistake. I knew I wasn't supposed to be there but I took advantage of the situation. I completed the course with honours and was promoted to corporal. The past seemed to be swept under the carpet in the Army's eyes, but not in mine.

I met a young private soldier and fell in love with her. Everything started to take shape again. The only one of four children who didn't have a family of his own was about to change. Leanne and I were together for about four months and were already talking about getting married and having children. We were in love and wanted to spend the rest of our lives together. The Army had other ideas. I was notified that I was being posted to Townsville. We tried to get her a posting up there as well, but there were no positions for her. She tried to get a discharge but was not allowed. The only option left was for me not to re-enlist and end my career. I was faced with a situation I didn't want to be in. I didn't want to make the choice between her and the Army, but I did. I threw away everything I had worked so hard to achieve for love. Only a couple of months later I found out that she had been seeing someone else. I was devastated. I packed up and went home to Bendigo. I drank heavily and started smoking dope again. I spent nearly every night in the pub with a mate with whom I shared a house.

Drinking took my mind off Leanne and eventually I had gone from being sad to being angry. I hated her for what she had taken away from me. Once again the booze had started to run my life. I tried to rejoin the Army but was told I could not because of drug allegations made against me. So I tried another option, the Army Reserve. This time I was successful. I was enlisted and employed as a full-time soldier at the Army Survey Regiment at Bendigo. I was still drinking, but only what I thought was in moderation. My posting at Bendigo was only for six months, and it gave me the edge I needed to try and re-enlist into the regular army again. It was then that I befriended a bloke in the local pub. He seemed like a decent enough sort of bloke and we got on pretty well. All of a sudden he was on charges of child pornography and other related charges. He asked me to lie to the police to get him off the charges. The police found out and had me wired to record the guy spilling his guts. He did, which meant that I had to go to court and testify against him. I was shit scared of this guy. He knew what I'd done and was making all sorts of threats against me. The police just kept on saying he was harmless and that he wouldn't do anything.

Who to tell?

It was then that things started to turn to shit for me. I drank heavily. At one point I was found asleep behind the local pub as drunk as a skunk. I smoked dope excessively. Every opportunity I could I would get off my face one way or another ... Everything just seemed to be happening and I didn't know how to deal with it. I didn't want to talk to my friends or family because they would look at me as a failure. After all, there I was at 26 years of age with nothing but an old car and only enough money to buy grog and smokes. I had nothing. I would go home of a night and just cry. I needed to talk to someone. I knew that. But who? Who would listen to me without saying 'It's easy, just get off the piss'. It was when I drank in the pub with a bloke and got pissed that I spilt my guts to him about nearly everything that was on my mind. It was then that I first told someone that I wanted to end this shitty life of mine. But who did I tell? A bloke I didn't even know and a bloke who ended up as full as a shit-carter's hat who didn't remember a word I'd said to him.

The following night I was back drinking at the same pub with a mate and two women. We drank until about 11 o'clock. We then decided we would go to a disco in the city about 5 km away. My housemate was also at the pub but decided he would stay there. I decided that I should get dressed up a bit, so I told them I would walk home and get changed and they could pick me up. Our house was only about metres from the pub, so off I went. I walked into the house and sat at the kitchen table. I didn't want to go to the disco and didn't want to do anything anymore. I walked into my mate's bedroom and found his shotgun in the cupboard. I then went out to the back shed where I knew he kept the ammo. I took two cartridges inside and loaded them into the gun. All this time, I was hoping that my friends would turn up and finally I would have to talk to them and tell them how I felt. But they didn't, they were too busy at the pub getting pissed. It was then that I sat down at the table and scribbled on a piece of paper 'Tell Mum and Dad that I'm sorry and I love them'. I put the gun between my legs and rested my chin on the barrel. I remember trembling as I slowly squeezed the trigger. Nothing happened. I had left the safety catch on the gun. I started crying and then removed the safety catch and pulled the trigger. As soon as I pulled the trigger I tried to pull my head out of the way but to no avail. I remember a bright orange flash, then a deafening blast in my ears. It was like slow motion as I fell to the floor.

I was lying on the floor for about a minute before I opened my eyes. I knew then that I wasn't dead but didn't know how long it was going to take. I lifted my head to see a large pool of blood getting bigger each second I laid there. It was at that moment I said to myself 'Fuck this, I don't want to die'. I crawled from the kitchen into the hallway and pulled the phone to the floor. I dialled 000 and asked for an ambulance. But something was wrong. They couldn't understand me and I became frustrated. Over and over again I tried to tell this bloke on the phone my address but he couldn't understand. Then finally I heard him say that someone would be there shortly. I was getting weak, and deep down, knew I was running out of time. I was losing too much blood and I knew it. Then I thought they would knock on the door and I would be unconscious and not hear them. With what strength I had left, I managed to open the front door and crawl outside. My mate turned up to pick me up and found me out the front. He ran inside and wrapped a towel around my face. Then I saw the flashing lights of the ambulance. I remember being put on the stretcher and going in the ambulance. I was getting weaker and the ringing in my ears started to go quiet. Then all of a sudden everything started to fade and the voices were going away. Regretfully, I thought I had succeeded and that it was over for me.

A minor hiccup

I woke up to see a man standing over me with a video camera. I didn't know where I was and I was scared. I looked around and saw lots of lights and people rushing around. I realised I was in a hospital so I relaxed and drifted off to sleep. I was unconscious for about two days. When I finally woke up, I remember trying to speak to a male nurse who was standing in front of me. I was trying to say something but nothing was coming out. He guided my hands towards my throat and told me I had a trachea insert in my throat to help me breathe. I was praying so hard that this was all some kind of hideous nightmare I was having, and at some point I would wake up and everything would be the way it should be. Over the next few days I was seen by many doctors. I was in and out of the operating theatre so many times that I lost count. For some reason I thought that things couldn't be that bad because I was so alert. I woke from one operation with a metal frame on my head. It was to keep what facial bones were left in place so they could try and piece me back together. I knew then that I was in bad shape. I lost any confidence I had of things going back to normal. They never would and I knew it. At that point, and for the first time in my life, I truly did not want to live. I had visions of being something like the 'elephant man'. Someone for people to stare at, someone for people to laugh at. I didn't want to go through it.

I communicated to people by using a pen and paper. My Mum and Dad were with me the whole time. I knew I loved them so much but couldn't understand why I put them through the hell I did ... I had seen many tears from Dad's eyes, tears I know I had caused and it hurt me. We spoke of things that we had never spoken of before. We became closer than we ever had before. Dad didn't care about what happened. He never asked why, he just looked ahead and spoke of all the things we could do. He reassured me that it was only a minor hiccup, and that I would get over it. I believed him and said to myself: 'I am going to beat this'. I had created some big hurdles that I was going to have to get over if I was to return to a normal life again. I knew that if I really wanted to I could. I knew that I was, for once, wholly responsible for my own actions. I knew the doctors were in control of what I would look like, but I was the one who was in control of whether I lived or died — and I wanted to live. I was no longer afraid of death. I had been there and I didn't like it one bit. I wanted so badly to live and try to make something out of nothing. I wanted to prove to everyone that I had made a terrible mistake, one which I would overcome.

Crunch time

Then it was crunch time. The sister-in-charge of the ward thought it was time I faced what I was dealing with. The constant dribble, the hole in my throat, the constant attention from nurses was all put before me. It is a moment I will never forget. She pulled the curtains around the bed and held a large mirror in front of me. I wept uncontrollably. My face was gone! I had my eyes and part of my nose and that was about it. My mouth and part of my tongue was gone. I had no jaw; nothing under my left eye; it was all gone. I was devastated. How could anyone repair something that was as bad as what I was looking at? I didn't want to look at it. I didn't want anyone else to look at it either. I demanded that the curtains remain drawn around me. I refused to see visitors except for my family. I was a monster, something you would see in a movie. I hated myself.

After a while that same nurse just walked up and pulled around the curtains. I was scribbling frantically about how much I hated her for what she had done. She then put the mirror in front of me and gave me a heap of dressings and told me I had to change my own dressings. I hated her even more. I refused to do it and so did they. After a time, the weight of dribbling saliva into the dressing was too much. I took the mirror and changed my dressing. The whole time, not once did I take any notice of the injuries. I looked at what I was doing and that was that. It became easier after that. I noticed that people were not looking at my injuries when they were talking to me. They were looking into my eyes. Then I had to convince the doctors that I was worth trying to fix up. I knew that if they thought I was just going to try what I did again, they would not bother doing a good job.

From then on, I only had one thing on my mind and that was to get fixed up, get out of hospital and get on with my life. Many of the nurses became counsellors. I had many issues I had to think about, like would I ever be loved by anyone. Would anyone ever see the love and passion I had to offer through the scars? Would anyone ever give me a job? How would I make a living? Would my family ever forgive me? Would I ever have a child of my own? Would people ever respect me, or would I just be thought of as a suicidal no-hoper? With the help of talking to all these people, it dawned on me that I was the one who had those answers. I spoke openly about where I was going and what I wanted from life. I set goals and I knew that if I wanted something badly enough I could have it. After all, I wanted to live so badly when I had seen that blood on the floor that I did survive; if I hadn't, then I would have just lay there and waited to die.

I stayed in hospital over 12 months. I made a lot of friends and it became my home. It was my shelter from the rest of the world. On some occasions I would go outside with friends, but couldn't wait to get back inside. The operations were still happening, and I was reassured that the worsening condition of my face was all part of the long-term result. The doctors had my trust — one in particular, Mr Ian Taylor at the Royal Melbourne Hospital. He seemed to take a particular interest in me. After many procedures and many skin grafts, the final major operation took place. With my hipbone grafted to my chin and balloons from America inserted into my neck it was D-Day. I woke to see a face again. It needed a bit of touching up, but it was there and it was mine. They stretched the skin over the chin so I could grow a beard. I was relatively normal again. Now it was time to go home and start again. Not to put the past behind me, but to learn from it and realise just how important I was to everyone who helped me overcome it.

The courage to talk

It is now 10 years later. I fell in love with a wonderful woman named Lyn. She would often visit me in hospital. She never offered me any sympathy, only encouragement. I didn't know then that it would be her who would see affection and not scars. She has three children from a previous marriage. I love those kids as if they were my own. I became a father to them and they too did not look at the scars but they looked beyond. They respect me for who I am and don't even asked what happened to me anymore. Lyn and I have had a child of our own too. She is a beautiful baby girl whom I love dearly. I gained qualifications in the earth-moving field. I travelled to Darwin and was employed not on the basis of what I looked like but the qualifications I held. I have gained employment easily and hope to start my own business in the near future.

Life is great now. Life was always great. I just needed to evaluate certain aspects of my life and redirect the paths I was taking. My biggest regret is that I failed to set positive goals and follow them through. I also regret not talking about my problems to those whom I knew would have listened — those who are not going to tell you what to do but offer positive advice. Had I done that, maybe the trauma I put myself and everyone I loved through may have been avoided. I was afraid of being labelled a 'looney'. I know now that I was not. I wish I had had the courage to talk instead of the courage to pull the trigger.

By the way, I have nothing but the utmost respect and admiration for Sister Lainie Anson of the Royal Melbourne Hospital. Without her, I would still be hiding behind curtains.

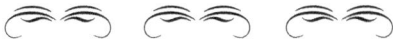

DIEGO'S COMMENTS ON TREVOR'S STORY

This is a tale of despair but also of courage. It is reassuring to know that the events that Trevor recounts happened ten years ago. This indicates that he has now 'metabolised' his past negative experiences, and the disconcerting roller coaster of emotions — I am ready to die, help me to live — has finally stopped, and in the best possible way.

Trevor contacted me via email — I have never met him personally. Though many other stories reach me through the Internet, Trevor's story is decidedly unusual and that is why I have included it.

Trevor presents as a fairly typical young man. He is young and wants to do something both manly and respected. What better than a job in the Army? However, it seems that he is not as strong and disciplined as 'good soldiers' need to be. In addition, Trevor picked up some bad habits from the Army, including alcohol and drugs. And, as many young men do, he starts to lose himself in pubs, dope and LSD. The slope soon becomes very slippery.

After these initial ups and downs, he meets a soldier-girl and falls in love with her. This brings some light to his darkening life, and Trevor adapts with enthusiasm to this new situation: he is ready to sacrifice his career and quit the Army, even though his relationship is only a few months old. But disillusionment awaits him — the love of his life has been seeing someone else. From stars to stables ...

Drugs and alcohol become centre stage again. They are not the right remedy for his anguish; he is aware of this. He would like to give vent to his anger and resentment, if only he knew how. But who can he talk to? And, after all, is it appropriate for a man (a soldier at that) to open up about such intimate issues, even worse, pangs of love?

So Trevor does not talk to anyone; actually, he ends up by befriending a 'bad guy', and thereby adding more stress and tension to his shaken life.

His description of his deadly attempt to end his young life comes across as rather 'dry', but it is in fact very true to life.

Readers might be puzzled by his apparent lack of premeditation or preparation for the fatal moment. He was heading to a disco and going home just for a quick change of clothes, so how likely is it that he would decide so suddenly? Well, throughout this book readers can see demonstrated that this is the way many suicides do actually happen. Most probably the idea of suicide was in Trevor's mind for quite some time, ready for enacting in a particular moment of despair. This is often the case — but not always. We learn from those who survived their suicide attempt (dead men don't speak; we have to rely on Trevor-like cases to know more about the suicidal process) that such ideation can become operational in the space of a few minutes, even seconds.

The ambivalence that Trevor describes during his suicide attempt is typical of most suicidal acts: he prepares to die but would like to be rescued by his friends.

The physical consequences of his suicide attempt are devastating, and of a severity certainly not common in suicide attempters. We know from literature that up to 7% of all attempters carry physical injuries as a consequence of their acts. David Lester, an English suicidologist, once proposed using photographs of injuries acquired from suicide attempts in public campaigns for suicide prevention. Lester took as his model the American actor Yul Brunner (a heavy smoker) who, when affected by lung cancer, altruistically allowed the image of his deteriorating body to be used for smoking prevention campaigns. Currently, cigarette packets carry as a deterrent images of human organs damaged by smoking. I would personally have reservations about such a project in the area of suicide, for a number of reasons; principally I would be concerned that people contemplating suicide would thereby be induced to do the 'job' well.

Trevor's 'rebirth' has not been smooth, it is a further roller coaster — expectations and hopes some days, and despair and the desire to die on other days. It is, however, a successful process, and the Trevor that emerges from the last line of his story is a much more mature man than the one we saw at the beginning of his story.

It is not the uniform that makes the man.

FOUR

Proxies

Anna's Story*

ear Diego,

As I sit here trying to recount my experience, I realise the strength I must have had to carry on and continue for so long without resolving the very issue that caused my suicide attempt at age 14. Twenty years on I sought help and was able to begin to overcome a life overshadowed by so many losses.

I now find myself still on the same journey — that of wanting to make a difference, but operating from a very different paradigm. Rather than needing to deflect from my own pain, I come from the space of having delved into the pain, accepting it and wanting to inspire others to see their own inner strength and capacity to change their own lives.

My name is Anna* and I was a victim of child sexual abuse from the age of five to the age of twelve. The perpetrators were neighbours, family friends and finally my grandfather. In all, I was abused by two women and three men. As with so many victims of such abuse, I suppressed the memories and told myself I was lucky that I was never penetrated. I grew up feeling 'dirty' and 'bad' and thinking that sex was wrong. I never dealt with the abuse, because I had rationalised that it was my fault — after all, I was the only common denominator. How could five adults be wrong?

---

* Anna's real name has been changed to protect the privacy of the contributor.

Unfortunately for me, it took a bad 13-year marriage and strained sexual relations within that marriage to finally force me to deal with an horrific chapter in my life. Through nine months of weekly counselling with a child sexual assault worker, I finally realised my suicide attempt at 14 was an attempt to stop the pain. Tragically, the suicide attempt promptly succeeded the death of my grandfather — the last perpetrator.

I now realise the day he died was the day that all my memories of the abuse came flooding back. My family's grief over his death served me little and caused me yet again to push memories behind. The unbearable pain I felt caused me to attempt to take my life, to end the suffering and the pain. The unsuccessful attempt resulted in little more than further pushing away the shame and guilt I felt. The litany of hospital social workers and youth workers I saw could not get to the bottom of my angst. They 'swallowed' my shallow reasoning that my attempt at suicide was because of a lack of freedom. I am most disheartened that no one could help me back then. No one could save me from two decades of self-criticism and an inability to take care of myself and meet my own needs and put myself first.

My first recollection of abuse was of the age of five. We lived in an apartment and the building's janitor would take me to school in the mornings. We had to cross a railroad track to get to the school and the janitor would hoist me onto his shoulder to get me across safely. The irony was that he used this opportunity to rob me of my innocence and would molest me on the way to school. I do remember sensing that something was wrong. However, being so young all I could articulate to my mother was that I didn't like the janitor and didn't want him to take me to school. My mother, who was working full time, said that it was too bad — he was doing her a favour by taking me to school and I had to live with it.

Little did she know what I had to live with! The clear message I got at such a young age was that my feelings did not matter and that my mother was not available to help me or even aware enough to question me further. This set a very dismal scene for subsequent experiences of abuse where I learned to suffer in silence. I don't remember when this abuse stopped. I only remember that there were other perpetrators and that the abuse did not stop.

The next lot of perpetrators were my neighbours — two sisters and a brother — they were different because I had fun with them. They would often invite me over to play. The sisters would ask me to hop into bed with them and made a game of making me touch their genitals. I am not sure what their brother did with me — I only recall him ejaculating once. At the time I didn't now what ejaculation was — it was much later that I realised what had happened. We migrated to Australia when I was seven, where we lived with my maternal grandfather for some time until my mother could get established. My mother bought an apartment near where my grandfather lived. She was doing shift work and had two jobs. I was often left on my own and regularly went to visit my grandfather, who took over where my other abusers left off. He molested me on a regular basis for several years.

I recall the confusion I felt, as I loved him and felt very close to him, but knew that what he was doing was wrong. He threatened me that if I ever told anyone what he was doing, they would never believe me and I would get into big trouble. I believed him and of course trusted him — at least he gave me attention and amidst the abuse was very kind to me. He stopped abusing me before my 12th birthday. Somehow I managed to block all the abuse out and was able to continue to have a relatively close relationship with him until the day he died — just before my 14th birthday.

Sunday 23 March, 1980

My recollections of my youth suicide attempt are like this. We received a phone call from the hospital to say that my grandfather had died. I knew when the phone rang what the news would be; I was stoic, numb to the grief around me. I had been fighting with my parents, because I wanted to go away with some friends and my parents would not let me. I was devastated that they would not let me go. That night I sat in my room feeling miserable, my life was unbearable. My relationship with my mother was tumultuous and I was distant to my stepfather. My eldest brother and sister-in-law were always there for me, but I felt such a burden on them — I couldn't keep running to them. I felt hopeless, helpless — so alone. I could not see a glimmer of hope, all I felt was despair.

I went to the bathroom in the garage where the medicine cabinet was; I grabbed a stack of my grandfather's prescription medication and went back to my room. I sat on my bed selecting the cocktail of pills that would end my life. I lay there confirming my decision with an arsenal of thoughts: 'I am hopeless, bad at school, I can't get on with my parents, I am a burden to my support people, I cannot bear another moment of this anguish. I can't cope anymore, I hate my life, I have nothing to live for'.

When my parents went to bed I went to the bathroom, locked the door, poured myself a glass of water, and began popping pills. I don't know how many I took, but I stopped only because the water was making me throw up. I went to bed and fell asleep. At some point in the night (about 3 a.m.), I woke up and started to walk to the bathroom but my legs gave way. I felt very drowsy but managed to get myself back up and dragged myself across the floor to the bathroom. I proceeded to take more pills, again stopping when I could not take any more water. I stumbled into bed and fell asleep straight away.

My parents woke me up to go to school — it was March 24 — my birthday. I got dressed, as if in slow motion, and waited on the lounge drowsily, my parents barely noticed. The phone rang — it was my sister-in-law ringing to sing me Happy Birthday. I got on the phone and after she sang she asked me how I was. My speech was slower than usual and she kept asking me 'What's the matter?'. I burst into tears and told her what I had done. She told me to stay home from school and sent my brother to take me to the local hospital. I told my parents I was feeling sick and that my brother would take me to the doctor.

My brother arrived; I had all but passed out — I couldn't walk. He had to carry me to the car. We arrived at the hospital and he carried me into casualty; someone saw me straight away. The doctor called it a 'cocktail OD', but it was too late to pump my stomach and I had to stay under observation overnight. I slept through most of the day and was visited by my brother and sister-in-law that night. My parents were angry with me and didn't come to visit.

The next day I was assigned a social worker who talked to me and decided that my attempt was related to my lack of freedom and bad relationship with my mother. I was placed in the care of my brother until I was relocated to a foster family. The social worker had initially taken me to group homes where I saw many homeless young people — they were so different to me, I was scared of them — they were far more streetwise. I explained to the social worker that I could not live in a group home and that I needed to be placed with a foster family. In August that year my nephew was born. It was the first time since my attempt that I understood the value of life, that you are born to live and that no matter how hard things get, life is far too precious to throw away because it's 'all too much'. The attempt was a definite cry for help that was left unanswered, but it gave me enough of a scare for me to realise that if I had been successful I would have never known my nephew and the love of a family who were doing their best. That year, although I was in Year 9, I chose to do work experience with a probation officer for Department of Child Services. Since then, my studies and career subsequently took the line of: 'How can I make a difference in this world?', 'How can I let people be heard?'

I am not sure what changed my mind — why I chose to live. I guess in the main, I realised that I was loved a great deal. In retrospect, going to the group homes and meeting 'streetwise' young people made me realise how sheltered and fortunate I had been. I did not display the anger I saw in their eyes and in their hearts — that emerged much later in my life. More importantly, I subconsciously chose to manage my anger, angst and pain in devoting myself to the injustices of others. After all, when you are consumed with the suffering of others you are able to deflect from your own. In fact, I realise now that I became a master at avoiding my pain by focusing on that of those less fortunate. My will to live arrived with a realisation that diversion was the best medicine for my condition. It did not happen consciously, so I can only imagine that someone 'up there' gave me the strength to carry on.

Moreover, the biggest gift in my life was meeting the counsellor who changed my life. She was a social worker specialising in child sexual assault and somehow she came into my life at the right time — a time when I was already on a journey of self-development. As misdirected as it was, it was a beginning of truly wanting to understand and change my life. She was extraordinary in helping me understand that the abuse I was subjected to was shocking, the fact that I was not penetrated was meaningless, the degree of abuse is relative. The abuse was not my fault — I did not ask for it and I did not perpetrate it. These things freed me from a life of self-blame, self-hate and an inability to realise that I could take charge of my own life and that I had the capacity to walk away from an abusive situation. The nine months I spent with her were the beginning of my healing and gave me the tools to make real changes in my behaviour in every aspect of my life.

Twenty years on

I am pleased to say that 20 years on I am getting my life together. I have realised that much of my behaviour in relating to others had been shaped by my childhood experiences as a victim of child sexual abuse. I realised that some positive things came out of those experiences — I am the strongest, most resilient and compassionate person I know. I am raising two beautiful children who have a mother who fiercely listens to protect them. I am far from perfect but, by God, I am willing to learn and grow and truly look at myself. I am learning to stand on my own two feet and to set clear boundaries in my work, with my family, friends and partner. I am proud of who I am and can see the boundless potential and determination I have to achieve peace with myself and with the world around me.

In light of the repeated abuse I experienced over seven years, I am amazed at how resilient and strong I was to have achieved so much. I know that many people do not have the courage to deal with their past, let alone have the tenacity to use their experience to make a difference in the life of others.

⤙⤙ ⤙⤙ ⤙⤙

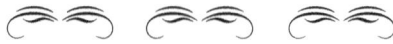

DIEGO'S COMMENTS ON ANNA'S STORY

Here a sensitive and intelligent young lady conveys to us one of the most painfully common antecedents to suicidal behaviours: sexual abuse. Though her abuse did not involve 'penetration', such a technicality should not induce any minimisation of utterly repugnant events. In addition, she relates how the abuse continued for many years, virtually her entire childhood, and came from different perpetrators, including a 'stable and reliable' and loved person, her grandfather.

Her descriptions are moving; and her narrative details the astonishment, confusion, embarrassment and blackmailing so frequently associated with the sexual abuse of minors. As a consequence of this most shocking abuse of trust, these victims are left incapable of forming normal relationships with their peers, unable to successfully engage in (voluntary) sexual behaviour and robbed of the resource to generate sufficient self-esteem.

People with a history of sexual abuse are frequently the clients of psychiatrists and psychotherapists, indicating just how deep and scarring this experience is, with its long-term consequences affecting the quality of all future relationships. In fact, these victims grow up lacking self-confidence and coping skills, and have little sense of control of their world or of their capacity to manage difficult situations. Such deficits may push them into dependency; however, they fear becoming dependent on others — they have learned that trust is foolish— for them, there is no one loyal and honest out there. Soon this lack of trust becomes inwardly directed: often people who have been subject to sexual abuse take on a mantle of guilt, they begin to perceive that they, themselves, are not trustable, that they are disloyal and dishonest. They have been corrupted and violated; they are not 'pure' anymore. Paradoxically, and sometimes stretching rationality to its extremes, a number of victims blame themselves for not having reacted effectively to their abuser, not having denounced the perpetrator when it happened, not having shouted their anger and resentment towards those around them who should have known what was happening and intervened to protect them. Instead, the victims feel that somehow they caused it; they let it happen and kept it silent.

Personally, I am not aware of any case of sexual abuse that does not have consequences for the sufferer. On the other hand, I have often heard — in astonishment — the minimising attitudes of the perpetrators of abuse, especially those who did not sexually penetrate their victims and who argue that there was no real physical violation; that, at worst, they only provoked some emotional turmoil.

I have heard such confessions from the abusers many times, and initially my reaction was to ask myself if these persons truly believed what they were saying or if their declarations were merely a form of alibi for themselves. My role is to help such people and not to condemn them; but I need to understand if they were aware of what they were doing and the consequences of their behaviour. In some cases I judge that the perpetrator was not aware of the damage of their actions, the blighting of a young life. They do not know it and surely they do not want to know it.

Some reveal more terrible confessions: that in turn, when they were young, they also were sexually abused by one of their parents, usually their father, or a relative or a close family friend, someone at any rate who benefited from the complete trust of the family. A few of these abusers are able to sense that the violence they perpetrated is related to the violations they received in their youth: becoming the 'active' perpetrator is a way of unconsciously, compensating for the damages suffered as a 'passive' victim.

In this story, the consequences of the abuse bring the victim to the point of self-destruction. There is much astute introspection in the narrative of our protagonist. It is of concern to realise that without the life-changing intervention of a good psychotherapist ('the biggest gift I have ever received in my life') things could have taken a very negative turn.

As in the case of the young woman of the following story ('The Box of Biscuits'), in 'Proxies', the protagonist's mother plays a central role (well, mothers are always 'central', for both good and the bad ...). Certainly, our young woman's tension with her mother, the lack of the natural father, and their immigration to Australia, all these elements contributed to render the surroundings in which she grew up into an environment that was rather unstable and risky, especially when she was required, too early, to cope with enormously disturbing and unsettling circumstances.

Our protagonist is today a woman and a mother. She is warm and competent and, largely, healed. She has started a career as counsellor. With all she has witnessed in her life, the least that can be said is that she is surely well positioned to understand human suffering.

FIVE

The Box of Biscuits
*Alessa's Story**

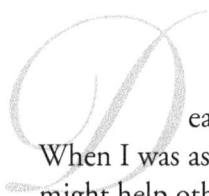

ear Diego,
When I was asked to tell my tale, my first thought was that it might help other people avoid making the same mistakes and to have a clearer understanding when certain things happen. Then I thought that it might help me too. I haven't done this sort of thing before, and the idea of putting pen to paper may even give me a few surprises. Perhaps I will recount something which is not true, to block any attempts at reconstruction of suffering, even though I now feel cold and hard, like a block of white marble.

Still here to tell the tale
I am now 33 years old. For at least 25 years my life has been hell, and it is merely by chance that I am still here to tell the tale. My name is Alessa*, which is clearly not my true name (although my real one is just as strange). I was born in Italy to a wealthy family (only in terms of money, though). My father was always at work, and naturally was never around. He went from one plane to the next and every so often would bring all sorts of people to our home by the sea (the representative house), and we had to be 'polite' to his guests. 'We', because I have a sister who is two years younger than me, but it is as

* Alessa's real name has been changed to protect the privacy of the contributor.

~ 71 ~

though I never had one, except for the problems she caused and the ritual family get-togethers.

My father was a handsome man, and still is. He no doubt had other women. I have always been convinced of this, and so has my mother. She was a beautiful woman too, only she never did anything. Her main occupation and uppermost worry was the summertime transfer to the seaside. It seemed that she had to organise an incredible transfer, whereas in reality the house had absolutely everything. I never really understood what there was to worry about. Every time, poor old Iseo (the summer house custodian) was forced to go backwards and forwards because mother had forgotten something, be it pins or pills. As far as I am aware, mum has always taken pills and has always seen doctors. My father used to accompany her to see the doctors, and then he stopped. He must have realised that Mother did not really have anything wrong with her at all, even though she appeared to suffer greatly. She spent many a day in bed, and often refused to see us. On those occasions, only Mirka (her former nanny) took care of her, and she didn't want dad to see her. I remember the corridor between the bedrooms at our town house being kept dark and Mirka telling us not to go there with our shoes on. Mother had to rest when, this happened and the light and noise bothered her. I can't say how long Mother's 'episodes' lasted. To me it seemed like always.

Once I accompanied Iseo to the airport to collect a doctor, a professor from Lausanne. My sister was at the international school full-time, and Father was away, Mirka could not leave Mother's bedroom, and so I was the one to go with Iseo. I clearly remember the professor. If I am not mistaken, Iseo had tried asking him something about the journey and received a monosyllabic reply. Two minutes later, you could have heard a pin drop in the car. The professor merely asked me whether I was Iseo's daughter, and when Iseo replied that I was Madam's daughter, he corrected him, saying that I was the patient's daughter. He looked at me in that strange way that was to become familiar a few years later. How I hate that expression. It's a combination of detached pity, false kindliness and interest in the 'microbe'. On the other hand, there is no way of showing a 'normal' face. Even if you succeeded, the damn doctor gets distracted, or thinks that you are acting, or that you can't possibly be really like that, as it is clear that if you are being treated by him, you must be stupid, or have a screw loose, or that you're different in some way. The professor was not a Swiss (even though to me he had a funny accent); he was an Italian who had gone to work in Lausanne. I don't remember how long he stayed at our house. I only know that my father was furious when he saw the bill and said that my mother must really be ill, because only a fool could be duped like that. And then he must be madder than her, as he was the one who paid in the end.

Every now and again, my mother would disappear, though it was not clear whether she went to her parents' house or to some clinic. When she returned, she seemed fine for a week or two, after which the usual saga would recommence. Dark corridors, ear plugs and so on. However incredible it may seem, my parents never separated, despite being so different from and intolerant of each other. The situation obviously didn't bother either of them all that much. My father could do what he wanted, as long as he paid doctors' bills and treatments; my mother could continue to do nothing, on the pretext of being ill. I don't believe I have many memories in which my mother was not crying. Her eyes had that faraway look, as though she were lost in a daydream, and were always sad, terribly sad.

An insatiable black hole

I was 10 years old when the ambulance drew up at the house for the first time. We were at the seaside, and strangely enough, were all at home ... parents and daughters, Mirka and Iseo. The ambulance had come for Mother. Mirka told me that mother was suffering from heat stroke, and that she was very weak and could not stand all that humidity. But when Father brought her home the following day, he left a light green card from the hospital on which the only thing I managed to read was 'gastric lavage'. As I was later to realise, this was followed by other attempts of suicide.

The worst episode was when I returned home for the Christmas holidays after having been sent to a convent boarding school. I was 15 years old. I had spent middle school with another order of nuns. My sister was also at boarding school, but in another town. She, too, was expected home that day. I now saw her so little that I didn't even know what hairstyle she had or how she dressed. I was laden with presents that Sister Maria had helped us get ready and was anxious to see what effect they would have. I had brought something for Mirka and Iseo too, and was ready to receive a hero's welcome. I knew that Father would soon be home. He always went to Frankfurt before Christmas and would come home with those spiced German biscuits that only he liked. I was more interested in the delightful biscuit tins, which I used for putting away photos, postcards and the like. I remember the scene as though it were yesterday. No one had opened the door to let me in. But I had not let that worry me too much. I was out of breath, full of bags and parcels, to the point that the taxi driver literally had to prop me up right to the front door, and I couldn't wait to present myself on the hall Bukhara as the most precious Christmas present of all. I had the keys and, after somehow getting up to the first floor, I had the impression that there was no one in.

It was four o'clock in the afternoon and pitch black. I dropped everything on the Bukhara, which was supposed to hold me like a queen, and began to wander round the house, calling Mother, Mirka and Iseo, one at a time. Strangely enough, Mirka and Iseo were not to be found. Mother was, unfortunately; and in a place she should never have been. I found her lying on the kitchen floor in a pool of blood. My heart stood still. I didn't react. On the contrary, the first thing I thought (of which I am very ashamed of now) was that the Christmas I had been so looking forward to was taking a completely different turn. Then, at last, I began to attend to my mother. It was as though she was asleep and I couldn't understand where all the blood was coming from. Her left arm was covered in it, her head tilted to one side, facing upwards with her eyes closed. The bread knife, the serrated one, was lying on top of the dishwasher.

I must have been paralysed for a few minutes. I couldn't distract myself from the sight before my eyes and do anything practical. Not for one minute did I think of going near my mother (I should have tried to find out whether she was dead!). Then I received what felt like an electric shock and my brain started to function once more. I called the emergency services, begging them to come quickly. I gave them my boarding school address but, fortunately, as we were the only ones in town with that surname (in addition to being rather well known), they got there just the same. The business of the wrong address has been plaguing me for years, especially after a stupid psychoanalyst told me that I probably hoped my mother would die. But let's take things one at a time, the wrong address story is not the most important thing. My mother was alive and she made it.

My sister arrived home laden with her well-wrapped presents and parcels just as they were taking Mother off to hospital. Mirka, as it happens, was already at the hospital: she had acquired cancer of the liver. At the beginning of February, she left us forever. Iseo had been sent to deliver some Christmas presents to a few families, as he did every year. Father arrived the following morning. He said he missed the flight and there had been no other way of getting back. Moreover, nobody knew how to contact him, as he never told anyone which hotel he was staying in.

We were only able to speak with mother on Boxing Day, and she seemed even more upset that usual. She kept crying and saying, 'Good God, what have I done! Good God, what have I done!'. Ludo, my sister, and I placed our presents on the bedside table and left the room dumbfounded, with Iseo leading us from behind like two robots. My father, after the first visit on Christmas Eve, shut himself into his study. On that occasion, we practically only saw him for Christmas dinner. He departed on New Year's Eve, early in the morning, leaving an envelope for each of us containing a very brief note in which he excused himself for his continuous business appointments, professed his love for us and left us a considerable amount of money. There was no mention of Mother.

Looking back to that period, I don't know what upset me more: the situation with my mother, or Father's behaviour. I can only say that a cold feeling came over me, which has not completely left me to this day. It was as though my body was an empty shell, or rather that my inner self had been swallowed up by a sort of insatiable black hole. The result was that I began to put on weight. The following Christmas I was almost 70 kg, 20 more than usual. I looked awful and the more I detested myself, the more I ate especially sweet things. I was capable of spending my entire pocket money in those days — during the ritual Sunday outing — on tubs of ice cream, biscuits and pastries, which I would then hide in my school bedroom.

That year, during the Christmas holidays, my mother had a psychiatrist come to the house under false pretences. She had passed him off as an old friend of the family, home for Christmas.

I had, however, smelt the rat almost immediately, both because I had learned to recognise his sort, through the ones who had come over to see Mother, and because I immediately recognised 'that' look. Moreover, Mother didn't have any 'family friends'; it was Father, if anyone, who had them.

When I confronted her, she desperately denied any involvement, but then told me that I had become a barrel and she was ashamed of me, and that no one would want me, nor would seek my company in that condition. To tell the truth, even at 70 kg I was the source of fun at school. Academically, I produced very poor results, but I was the leader of all the girls and nothing happened or was organised without my consent. Even the 'smoking sessions' (pot, of course) were managed with scientific efficiency. What I can't understand though, is how the nuns didn't recognise the smell of grass!

The happiest day of my life

That year was of paramount importance in my life. While I was at home for Easter, I met at a disco 'the love of my life', who was able to do much more for me than any psychiatrist and his advice. In less than six months I had returned to my former weight and wasn't looking bad at all. When I saw my man during the following Christmas holidays, he didn't even recognise me, but wanted me straight away. I became pregnant at 17, and at 18 naturally was married in a church, dressed in white, with a whole host of people whom I had neither seen before nor heard of. They were mainly friends of my father, people who were only able to gift silver, both modern and antique, of every style. So much so that it filled the whole library, living room and (playing) card room. My husband had diligently taken it upon himself to stick labels with the giver's name on each item, as otherwise it would have been impossible to make any attempt to thank the various people. My parents behaved according to cliché: Mother with her faraway look and tearful eyes (you could have mistaken her for being moved), and Father, with his managerial appearance and wit, true to any board meeting. It was the happiest day of my life. I was totally oblivious to any practical or essential problem connected with the new life which lay ahead. What did I need to worry about? I was 18 years old, expecting a baby, attractive; my friends envied me and I didn't care one little bit about leaving school. I had married the most handsome man in the world. What more could I want?

At this point, I have not yet spoken about my husband. I must admit that even now it is not easy to talk about him. In any event he was good-looking, very good-looking. He was 12 years older than me, and worked in the clothing industry at the time. He had a factory with a friend of his that produced jeans and T-shirts, and he travelled a lot for work, like my father. He had a yellow Ferrari and an enormous black motorbike, and when I mounted it (like on our wedding day) I felt I was driving through paradise. I must have been totally 'off my head' at the time. Father had bought us a country house as a wedding present. It was in fact an 18th century residence with a series of barchessas and secular magnolias, seven kilometres from the town. I didn't even know he had bought it, nor, to tell the truth, did I know how much money my father possessed nor less still how he made it. Neither then nor now.

We spent our honeymoon in Mauritius. We went to the airport by motorbike, in our wedding attire. Some friends of my husband followed us in a car with a change of clothes and our luggage. It was like a dream, the happiest moment of my life. My tummy was not so big and he wanted to make love continually.

One day, we sniffed coke (cocaine) together. He insisted, saying that the baby was too big for anything to happen to him. After this time however, I didn't want to do it anymore. I already felt high with all the joy and I felt I didn't need anything else. He, instead, began taking it practically every day. He kept the powder in his shaving brush handle, saying that no one would have ever found it there. His supplier friend from London had travelled in every corner of the world with a similar sort of toilet bag, avoiding every type of control.

Niki (the false nickname I am giving to my husband) was self-assured. He had a roughish arrogance which would have made even the most prudish of my nuns blush. Oh Niki, Niki, how deeply I loved you! And how different things would have been if you had really been what I thought you were. Shortly afterwards, as quickly as the gates of heaven had opened, I just as rapidly fell into the depths of hell.

Into the depths

I had my first inklings when we returned home. The villa was splendid, a dream house, but inside here was only silverware, a few pictures, a couple of vases and a expensive coffee maker machine; the most prosaic gift, but also the only one which I could use in some way. All the furniture was to be bought, but I was unable to make decisions on my own. I was only a pregnant girl with no domestic skills. Niki would help me with the buying, I thought. And Iseo would certainly have aided me in everyday affairs. But that's not how it went. When Mirka died, Mother had not employed anyone else. She had even started doing the ironing herself, while Iseo did the cooking. When I called my mother from the airport to ask whether she had seen to anything (the beds, for example) and whether I could borrow Iseo for a while, she replied and I clearly remember her words — that borrowing Iseo was out of the question and that we could spend that night at the nearby hotel. I could have always asked Niki's family — who were all well off — to give us a hand. Niki's family, alas, had never lifted a finger, not even after the birth of Benedict. As for Niki, he left for London three days later. On business, he said. Even though I felt like someone who has been beaten around the head, I didn't lose heart. We did have a telephone and I began calling a few ex-school friends for advice. I wanted to show Niki that I could survive on my own and that he hadn't married a silly little goose. I wanted him to be proud of me.

To surprise him on his return, I asked Clara, a friend of mine who had started university that year, to come with me to buy some furniture. I almost emptied two shops. Father was paying. Three days later, I had a bedroom, sofas, dining table and chairs, a kitchen with a large fridge (the one which makes ice cubes: I had always fancied one), a television, vacuum cleaner and bathroom accessories. Basically, we could start living. I had also bought an *Artusi's* book for doing the cooking (Clara said it was the ultimate!). I had just spent enough to fit out a regiment. I later realised that I didn't understand a thing about the *Artusi*. So I phoned Iseo to get him to explain how to make spaghetti and roast chicken (I knew absolutely nothing).

Niki came home at dinnertime later than expected. He must have been high on coke. Immediately he made a scene about the furniture I had bought. He hated modern furniture and didn't want it in his house. With his eye's bulging out of his head, he practically destroyed the double bed, throwing the mattresses out the first floor window. In the meantime, I overcooked the spaghetti, which I tried to synchronise with Niki's return. In the kitchen, my husband, the most charming man in the world, slapped me so hard that I ended up sitting on the floor with my back against my coveted new fridge. Then he left, apparently pleased with his work. I decided to sleep on the sofa.

The following morning, I left the country for my parent's house, with worrying pains deep down in my tummy. Niki's scene had shocked and stunned me and I felt totally humiliated. However, I decided to put up a fight — but against whom? Niki had disappeared. At his home nobody knew where he had gone, nor at his office.

Benedict

Just over two months later, Benedict was born. He had Down's syndrome, yes, Down's syndrome! The slight form, according to that brazen-faced doctor at the clinic, but mongoloid just the same. They let me see him after two days. He didn't seem abnormal to me; but the nurse indicated his eyes and hands. She told me that he would have been a very affectionate child and that I would have loved him dearly. The bitch! It was as if she was talking to living death and I simply wasn't there anymore. I only know that I must have really been crazy, because I kept calling for my father.

After what must have been days, I woke up in a different clinic. My husband was there, in his god-like beauty, sitting among what seemed to me like pink cushions. I would have liked to have burst into tears and thrown my arms around him; after which I probably would have shouted at him and given vent to all my rage. However, I was unable to do either. My tongue was stuck in my mouth. My lips may have opened just slightly, and I was certainly unable to move my arms. Niki must have noticed because he stood up and came, towards me, but I couldn't understand what he was saying. Maybe there was someone else in the room too, but I drifted off again.

I spent six months in that clinic. I was angry, depressed, psychotic, and mad. 'Post-partum depression', diagnosed the Swiss professor, who had come back on the scene, with that face like a goldfish in a pond. I wanted to know about my child. He was well, I was told, and had been living at my parent's house. I, too, went to stay at my parents'. Every day a psychiatrist from the clinic came to see me and made me take enormous quantities of drugs. That was fine by me. The only thing I wanted to do was sleep, for as long as possible. When I was able to reason more clearly, I realised that something had changed at home. My father was home more than usual; but the greater change was in my mother, who seemed like a normal person, no longer a human larva. Benedict was well but his mongolism was now evident. Also evident was the fact that the new climate at home was all thanks to him.

Nobody wanted to tell me anything about Niki. Was he such a monster that he couldn't find time to visit his son? I called Clara and at last found out that Niki had been caught by the Spanish police, he had been in prison over there for three months, and then extradited. His car was found loaded with drugs, especially cocaine. Everyone in town was talking about it as it was in all the papers. A great scandal! I told my mother that I knew everything, and that we could talk openly about it. She told me that there was nothing to tell and that the only thing to do, as soon as I was better, was to file for separation. There was to be no more mention of his name in that house. And while we were on the subject, I might as well have known the rest: that Ludo had been expelled from school because she had been found taking drugs in the toilets. She was now enrolled at a private institute to enable her to finish high school and was living with Mother's sister, Aunt Erminia. From one catastrophe to the next, there was no doubt! And to think that less than a year ago, I had felt like I was in seventh heaven.

The psychiatrist who never stopped coming

Shortly afterwards, since I had started to get used to my new family life, I began to feel ill again. I couldn't sleep and had started talking to the television, or rather I thought the television was telling me how to behave at home, what I had to wear, etcetera. The psychiatrist, who never stopped coming to visit me at home, decided to admit me to hospital in the Department of Psychiatry. He felt I was too serious to go back to the ward I had been in previously. I left hospital labelled schizophrenic: they gave me a jab every 15 days (which killed me!) and I took drugs which made me as lucid as a drunkard and as agile as someone inside a diving suit! As soon as I stopped feeling controlled, I went back on to dope — like Ludo. And like Clara, who had wanted to give me a little relief, starting me off on that new life.

In a short time, I had gone through the basic steps: I became addicted, got involved in dealing, stole and had trouble with the law. I became as thin as a pin, with awful, grey skin and lank hair. The Swiss professor reappeared. He opted for psychoanalysis, for which I had no desire. They ended up sending me to someone who looked like a priest with stigmata. Strike me dead if he looked me once in the face! I could have taken a tape-recording with me and slept through the session, without him even noticing. He always wore the same Austrian-style grey jumper with bone buttons. There was a faint smell of baby poo in the room. Fortunately, after a short while I was so bad that I had to go back into hospital and never saw the 'priest' again. They took me back to the Department of Psychiatry, but after a few days with the usual horse therapies, my father (incredibly) reappeared with another psychiatrist who wasn't half bad (I still took an interest in men now and then). He convinced the doctors to allow me to be admitted to a clinic in Rome and would accompany me and present my case (what could he know about me?). I really did go to Rome, where they gave me six electroshocks and lithium and I returned home two months later.

I was no longer schizophrenic. I was now 'schizoaffective', and slightly drug dependent — thanks to them. At home I was taken into the care of a kind, dynamic psychiatrist. He helped me to give away drugs, even though it wasn't at all easy. Every now and again, some pusher would rear his ugly head and a couple of rogues had tried to involve me in a trial or two. Father probably sorted things out, with some money.

Time to die?

For a few years I was reasonably well. I had also started working as a secretary in one of Father's companies. Occasionally he took me on business trips with him. I didn't take any care of Benedict; he didn't even call me Mummy. My mother was always the one who looked after him (her depression had stopped), together with a teacher who lived in. My sister Ludo was living in a community in Tuscany and wanted to marry a guy she had met there. My parents now seemed capable of accepting anything life put to them, like a natural need to atone for their forefathers' errors.

That is, until three years ago. It was almost Easter time when I decided it was time to die. I must say it happened all of a sudden. Or rather, I had contemplated it on numerous occasions, but to be honest, the thought hadn't been in my mind for a while. I had got into a reasonable routine: I had my job (with rather flexible hours), Benedict seemed to be sorted out (I felt very guilty towards him even though I knew I couldn't have coped with anything different), my parents talked to each other like never before, I even had a few friends, and my psychiatrist was pleased with me; the blood lithium levels were almost in order and I went to my fortnightly appointments regularly.

Basically, I wasn't doing so badly. Yet that Saturday afternoon I decided that my hour had come, that the time was right, and that there was no point in going on. That morning I had seen my psychiatrist, who had complimented me on my strict adherence to the therapy (lithium and a sedative in the evening). I had eaten hurriedly because I felt very sleepy and wanted to go to bed. Before going to my room, I had tried teaching a new song to Benedict. My mother had scolded me for spending so little time with him (but what would she have done otherwise?). Then, at last, I went to my bedroom. I got into bed but couldn't sleep. I felt unnerved and was rather surprised that my sleepiness had passed so quickly. I began to turn out the wardrobe, where I found a couple of those tins of the Schmidt biscuits Father liked so much. I looked inside. Among old souvenirs I came upon a letter which I had written to my mother from boarding school immediately after the Christmas when I found her lying on the kitchen floor. I was suddenly overcome by the conviction that everything had been horrible and that I could no longer do anything with passion or hope. I was overcome by a sense of suffocating anxiety. The colours around me changed. I seemed to be surrounded by greyness (my bedroom was very colourful); at most I could see various shades of grey. My head was spinning and I felt I couldn't breathe anymore. A lump rose in my throat as though I was being strangled. Without realising what I was doing, I was down in the laundry. Two bottles of stain remover came into view ...

I woke up, still in this world, after being in a coma for three weeks. It was a miracle, they told me. I wasn't too sure about the 'miracle', because then another cavalry began: rehabilitation, physiotherapy, speech therapy, etcetera, and etcetera. In addition, I had a hole at the base of my throat (from the tracheotomy). My mother had a cameo as big as a clock ready for me, which had been a present from Grandma Vittoria. Everyone was very kind to me and lots of people came to see me, including my psychiatrist (who had been informed by my mother). Many school friends came too, and I felt alive again, cleaned of an inner filth which had been accumulating and accumulating to the point of suffocation. And now that dirt was gone, I felt unburdened and ready to retrieve, both physically and mentally, everything that was in my power to recuperate. I stayed in hospital for six months. When I left I could speak almost perfectly and limped only slightly on the right leg. My morale, however, was fully recovered.

Looking back, and I still don't understand why, I felt I have paid my debt with life and I am well. At times I even feel rather superior. I don't think I'm giving myself airs; it's just the way I feel.

Diego, I now discover that I have very willingly made all these notes. It has taken me an entire afternoon of effortless writing. I don't know whether what I have said may interest anyone or help them in any way. What I do know is that my life is not and will not be easy. But feel assured that the hell I have gone through will not be coming back — ever again. And that, whatever terrible thing may still happen to me, nothing and nobody can send me back down to the previous depths — ever again. Take Alessa's word for it!

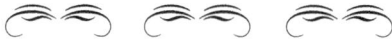

Diego's comments on Alessa's story

Alessa's story could rival the plot for a movie, it is so rich, and her voice so fresh in its telling.

Alessa would seem set to lead a charmed life — a beautiful young lady, and from a very wealthy family. However, life often teaches that such bounty does not automatically bring happiness, especially for those generations who haven't built the wealth from which they benefit. Alessa is no exception.

From her teens, our protagonist had problems in finding her place. It seems impossible for her to live a normal life; reality is too stark. Though on the surface she has everything that she can materially need, she knows that the life she is living does not belong to her. She must become addicted to dreams to make her reality bearable: otherwise the harsh facts of being uncherished and invisible are too painful to bear.

The suffocating figure of her mother takes the central role in this story. Marrying a handsome and successful man, but soon put aside by him, the mother adopts the sick role, not only to survive, but also to fight back: dark corridors, absolute noise prohibition, expensive doctors and therapies, are powerful weapons with which to express her aggression towards her husband, who has relegated her to a secondary role in his shining life of first-class travel, VIP cultivation and, presumably, plenty of beautiful women.

Alessa's mother seems completely inept; even the most trivial activity, like moving to their summer house, appears as an insurmountable obstacle. She is a mother who teaches her daughter that a suicide attempt is an effective way to be 'seen' and 'heard'. From the narrative it appears that her attempts were just that — attempts, only — judging by the setting for each. Though she was dicing with death, she was likely to be found in enough time. And if the suicide attempt was not 'successful', then usually she could wreak havoc in other ways, like being discovered unconscious during Christmas celebrations: her attempt at ruining the Christmas holidays for her family was certainly a success.

Alessa's mother has, like Alessa, retreated to a dream world. She completely neglects her children, ignoring their most basic needs and barely registering that her daughter is getting married. Ominously, she starts to take an interest in her daughter only when Alessa seems to be unwell: for her daughter's weight problems she arranges a visit with the very costly Swiss specialist (duplicitously disguised as a family friend); and later, she is probably behind Alessa's admission to the private clinic in Rome. But, surprisingly, she rehabilitates herself (in all senses) by taking care of Benedict, Alessa's child, who has Down syndrome.

As fate would have it, Alessa becomes much sicker than her mother, beset by a spate of ills: bulimia and postnatal depression, drug addiction, and finally 'schizoaffective' disorder. She rivals her mother in the severity of her psychiatric disorders. And, again like her mother, married to a handsome and successful man, she is cast off in her turn — even more rapidly than her father had cast off her mother. Life has dealt her severe blows. The fairy tale has ended, and on reading a letter that she had written to her mother some time before (and never posted? or received back marked 'Return to sender'?), too many horrible memories surface, and she impulsively decides to put a permanent end to her misery.

Fortunately she is granted another chance to live. When Alessa awakes from coma, it is an actual re-birth. Experiencing death so intimately has left her with the conviction that she is destined to live. She feels extraordinary, and as though she has now paid for all the mistakes she has made in life. The last paragraph of her story shines with determination and strength never possessed before. Her last sentence is a real *coup de theatre*: to give her word by using a pseudonym cannot be taken too seriously. However, her storytelling skills are evident, and this may have induced her, Stephen King-like, to set up a grand finale.

It is now many years later, and Alessa is alive and very well. Believe you me.

SIX

My Beautiful Grapes

Sergio's Story *

Dear Diego,

People are hesitant to believe my story. They think I'm trying to kid them, and they ask about the true cause of my limp. But then my eyes tell them that, incredibly, what I say is true, and I can see a kind of genuine admiration in their faces. No, it is probably not admiration, but a sort of sympathetic understanding of what has evidently been a tormented trip to expiation. And they are happy for me. I can see that.

My tallest silo

On the 21st of September, some years ago, I tremblingly climbed the stairs of my tallest silo. I looked at the world around me for the last time, through eyes full of tears. I made a deep sigh, my lungs echoing my despair. And I jumped off.

I could not make it anymore. Life had nothing to say and nothing to give to me anymore. I had no curiosity to anything, anymore. All I had was emptiness, darkness, and total disconnection.

I was living with my wife and my youngest son, who had been crippled after an accident with a tractor at the age of 12. He is the last of six children; he is the only one not married and living independently. None of them wanted to do my

* Sergio's real name has been changed to protect the privacy of the contributor.

job. I am a peasant. The eldest of them works in a bank, another runs a shoe shop in the city, and the other son is a policeman. My two daughters have two and three children, respectively, and it is their job to take care of them.

I should not have let my son drive the tractor at that age. I have never forgiven myself for it. Not even my wife has forgiven me, I am sure of that. Of course, she has always spoken contrary to this, but that doesn't matter. She too was born and raised in the countryside, but in those days there were very few tractors; oxen and horses were mostly used. Tractors were a luxury item for a few people. Anyway, my wife is right when she says that a lot of accidents, big or small, may happen when working in agriculture. And, unfortunately, this happened to my son.

He started, driving tractors, with me beside him, when he was two years old. He was a quick learner, with a great passion for doing that. The day it happened, he had just started ploughing a field of corn. He was driving too close to the edge of a small irrigation canal and the edge collapsed. The tractor rolled over; it was a miracle my son survived. However, from his right hip down he was literally in pieces.

I travelled the world to find him the best surgeons and the best therapies. After a number of interventions his right leg remained permanently rigid and still today he cannot flex it at all. He is as beautiful as an angel, his eyes as blue as the sky, but he will never find a woman, I am sure of that. People are pretty cruel about these things.

From that day on, I could not find peace in any way. My life became a nightmare: I had so much love for my land and my cattle before, and afterward I had so much hate.

I lived that way for more than five years, without joy for anything or anybody. I could not make love to my wife anymore. I kept working because we needed to earn a living, but I just did the minimum, only those things I could not avoid doing. In my life there were no seasons anymore, no sun anymore. I didn't feel the difference between warm and cold. My wife had to give me instructions on what to wear, and I simply obeyed her, without saying a word. I thought I had no right to talk; I didn't deserve any joy.

The only thing a sensible man had to do, I said to myself, was to die. It was me who encouraged my son to drive that damned tractor, and it was me who needed to pay for the consequences.

Peasants don't know much about what happens in the world. They don't like to talk too much. I had made a terrible mistake and nobody had yet punished me for it, but I knew that everybody considered me guilty for what had happened. I could read it on the faces of everybody, even of those whom I didn't know personally.

Destiny

I made every effort to convince myself that accidents may happen to everybody, even the most prudent ones. I tried to pretend that life could continue as before, had to continue as before. Elena, my wife, continuously warned me not to torment myself. Destiny had decided it to be that way, she said, and I had to stop thinking that I was the responsible for what had happened. I could not listen to those remarks. My youngest brother had incurred a similar accident, but his tractor was bigger, it had a cabin, and he remained trapped inside it with no wounds, until someone came to rescue him.

I should have learned from his experience, it should have been very clear in my mind. My son never said anything to me about the accident, but I thought I could read inside him what he was feeling. It would have been much better if he had shouted his anger out, I would have certainly felt relieved. But he said nothing, not a single word. Beautiful like the sun, he had his whole life in front of him. Me, I was not even able to raise children anymore. And now I was old and without a future to look forward to. I was someone stealing the bread that should go to the others. Why was I living?

Once my wife wanted to take me to our family doctor. I never liked that man, and going there was just a waste of time. He asked me how I felt, and I said OK. What was the problem then? And my wife intervened to explain what had happened, but of course he knew everything, since he was also my son's physician. He asked me if I felt depressed. Honestly, I could not say if, at that time, I really knew the meaning of the word 'depressed'. I answered asking him how he would have felt, had he incurred the same experience. He said that he understood my situation perfectly; but I had to try not to become ill because of it.

I didn't like that man because he didn't look at you when he asked you a question. I wonder how it is possible to be a doctor and treat people that way. How is it possible to understand that someone is sick if you do not even look at him or her? Then he asked my wife if there were cases of depression or other mental disorders in my family. When my wife started answering no, that she was not aware of any troubles of that kind in my family, I walked away from the doctor's surgery.

Once out, I cursed at my wife for that incredible waste of time. I remember that she replied to me that had I continued with that stupid behaviour, she would have become the first case of known madness in my family. I was rendering her life a hell, she said. What happened to us was not the worst misfortune, there were many real tragedies around, she kept saying. Her sister, for example, had lost a son in a road accident a few years before, and she had restarted her life with more courage and faith than ever. I have never had any faith, and I didn't get on very well with priests, maybe even worse than with doctors. My wife had to stop it, then.

Out of my role

After that argument, there were many months of complete silence. Maybe we were silent for more than an entire year. Then came the time for me to climb to the top of the silo.

In the preceding months the sense of oppression, pain, and guilt were becoming unbearable. I could only sleep for a few hours a night. My wife realised this, but when she tried to ask me why I couldn't sleep, I'd pretend to be asleep. Furthermore, I had started drinking much more than usual. I must admit that it helped me to find some momentary relief. My wife complained a lot about it: 'You'll end up like your father, he couldn't distinguish days from nights anymore, and became as nasty as a beast'. She also added that she would never accept a beating like my mother had received from my father. She would have eventually run away, should this have ever happened. In fact her words irritated me more than the awareness of my over-drinking, but I never ever thought to physically abuse her. I was fully aware that it was Elena who was running the family. I, instead, was totally out of my role and useless for people.

I loved to drink my own wine, the one we made. It gave me a special satisfaction. I used to merge the Merlot grapes with the Cabernet Frank in equal parts, and even if it was wine from the plains and not from the hills, it was very good nevertheless. It was my wine, and I always made it by myself ever since my father taught me how. I usually sold most of my production to the corporation of vineyards but kept 300 litres for our family use. I didn't put any preservatives in the wine, not even the bisulfite. It lasted in that way more or less 1 year, but it was honest and a good wine. In my opinion, it was the best of all. It was unmatchable with any other. I also produced white wine, some pinot and some tokai, but I never was one for white wines, I really didn't like them much. Consequently, I saved approximately 100 litres of it for the family, and the remainder was for sale. White wine is for women, my father used to say.

On that day in September we had already started harvesting the white grapes. It was an exceptional year. It rained and was sunny and dry on the right days, and the grapes were of a very good grade and were extremely abundant. But to me, it didn't matter anymore. My son, my crippled son, would take care of it. He knew very well how to manage it.

That cement silo is approximately 10 metres high. A bit behind the house, on the same side as my grapes, it was the first of the cement silos built around here. Built in two separate sections both 5 metres high, it is roughly 3 metres in diameter. When I bought it, I certainly did not think that one day I could use it for such a purpose.

Well, that day I climbed the silo's stairs around seven in the morning. The sun was already warm and shining. In the countryside people normally wake up very early. That night I could not sleep for a minute.

I cannot remember everything of that day, but I surely made a walk around the house, I saw my wife feeding the dogs and then going inside again. It took me quite a while to climb the stairs because I was shaking strongly and crying. Once over the roof of the silo I thought that all my pains were going to finish soon. My wife and my son would have had enough to live on. All my other children didn't need me anymore. They would have understood and forgiven me.

Joy unrestrainable

But then something happened, something really incredible. When I jumped off, I immediately thought that I did not want to die. I perfectly remember my dogs barking, I saw my grapes inundated by the sunlight, and my fields of corn recently threshed. In a short while also my red grapes should have been harvested. And then it came to my mind, all the energy and effort that I put into that property during my entire life. I rebuilt the old house, reclaimed the old marsh around the drain, added more than 30 hectares to those that my father had left to me. That property was everything to me and, honestly, was not bad at all. Maybe I could be useful again. In that precise moment I wanted to live, with all of my being.

But to die, I began my fall face down. Now I had to try to redirect my body. If I succeeded, I thought that, maybe by landing on my feet, I could eventually survive. And this was the case. I landed with my feet and legs first, rolling immediately aside, and amortising as much as I could of the terrible impact with the soil. The pain was even more violent than what I had imagined, but my joy was unrestrainable. I screamed, both for physical pain and happiness. My heels had gone, but the rest of my body was alive and well! Actually: freed and reinstituted to life.

My wife arrived immediately; she very clearly understood what was going on. I saw my son arriving from two parallel lines of grapes. He was limping like a mad horse, but in his way running, and fast. Well, from now on I will be destined to limp for the rest of my life, but I am also happier, certainly much happier than I was before.

I underwent a number of operations. My heels are of titanium now. I started moving the first steps in my new life after approximately three months. And, I swear, these really were the initial steps in my new life. A newborn of more than 60, inside I felt the enthusiasm of an adolescent.

I wanted to die, but at maybe 7 to 8 metres from death I changed my mind, and by a miracle I just managed to survive. Now, I am immensely happy for this. It doesn't matter if I'll be limping for the rest of my life. I'll still make a great wine anyway.

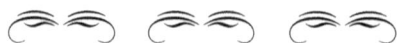

DIEGO'S COMMENTS ON SERGIO'S STORY

I was profoundly moved by this good man's story. During my career, I have known of such reverses: a sudden change of mind during the actual course of a suicide,[1] but nothing quite like this. There are in the literature, however, many such examples; the most recent I read is in the *Australian and New Zealand Journal of Psychiatry* (Cheah et al., 2008, pp. 544–546) and describes a young man's jump from a bridge, 49 metres above the water, of his change of mind during the fall and assumption of the 'pin drop' position. He survived with a few bruises.

This story is disarmingly simple. A hardworking farmer, a decent father and husband, and strongly involved in the success of all his children, is haunted by his guilt at having permitted his son, then aged 12, to drive his tractor. The tractor flipped over, leaving his son crippled forever. The farmer's mind returns again and again to this tragedy until he can't bear it anymore, and seeks to end his own life.

The 'hated' family general practitioner has surely pinpointed the nature and the severity of this man's suffering. However, the GP would have avoided mentioning the possibility of further help (via a psychiatrist — which would have undoubtedly been refused by the farmer) in order to maintain some bond with his patient. A forced admission to hospital would also have been seen as punitive, too hard to be explored. A GP in rural areas usually knows his patients very well: tough people, communicating only the essentials, secretive about their feelings or struggles, more comfortable with their countryside than with the company of other folks; deliberate people who have learned not to overly rejoice in a good harvest as the next might be wiped out.

Our farmer did his best, in the only way that he knew. He continued working and pretending he was able to sleep (thereby shielding his wife from worry). He did not question why his son (still as beautiful as an angel, but so crippled) was not shouting imprecations against him. It seems that the boy blamed himself rather than his father for the accident — it was evident that the farmer did not ever consider this reading of the facts.

So went the years, until, with the vulnerability of older age, and the false consolation of his wine, our protagonist set the circumstances for his prevailing mood to deepen and become acutely black and hopeless. Alcohol still remains the number one trigger in suicidal behaviours, even if it is, like our farmer's wine, of great quality.[2]

Perhaps his deterioration was also a consequence of other factors, derived from his style of coping: uncomplaining, silent, hard working; and unable to seek the solace of his wife, or, especially, of his injured son. In this way five long years wear by; then alcohol fuels his acceleration towards the epilogue.

His pride, for all his life, had been located in the simple things: he had improved and enlarged the property, the legacy passed down from his father into his care; modernised it and managed his stock effectively, and he gloried in his beautiful grapes. He was enfolded and comforted by his daily routine. And his beautiful family, of course.

It is with these images — filtered through a veil of tears — which the farmer jumps off the silo. Then, suddenly, a dramatic transformation occurs. There is no time for him to try to understand what has provoked a change of mind, but now the farmer desperately wants to live. Now he concentrates on changing the position of his body to avoid falling with his head first. Despite his age, he is still a strong man and agile enough to succeed in his intent. Heels and ankles are broken to pieces but his life is saved. He immediately understands that a new man has been generated by this deadly fall. He has passed a crucial test; his guilt is finally atoned.

The farmer limps more visibly than his son these days. His walking is difficult; his steps are slow and visibly tiring. But his soul has returned, and he has no hesitation to revealing himself to other, no hesitation in describing what happened. His wife says that he has become almost talkative!

In front of me I have a man who is smiling and whose eyes are lit with pride. Something heroic, maybe ...

Notes

1 For example, people overdosing with drugs but then calling the ambulance; others starting to gas themselves inside the car and midway opening the door.

2 A cautionary aside: addiction to alcohol ruins lives; it brings numbness, demotivation, loss of credibility, loss of job, relationship breakdowns, violence, and isolation, not to mention malnourishment and physical illnesses. Depression soon follows as a response to the first difficulties and failures. To cope with these, more alcohol is needed: and for a few hours it relieves anxiety and picks up mood. But then, like the true depressant it is, more anxiety and more depression arrives. The circle has closed.

SEVEN

The Missed Concert
Sandro's Story*

ear Diego,
It 'takes all sorts'; I know, so I feel privileged to be included in this collection.

Four years ago, I considered my life was finished. I had lost my job and I had lost my wife, the woman with whom I was deeply in love. She was seeing another man, not because she really cared for him, but because she couldn't handle life with me anymore. She was probably right; I was and still am a rather difficult person. But I have paid a heavy price, as this written record shows.

A career in the making

I was a pianist, and a very isolated individual, with very few acquaintances and virtually no friends at all. The only son of a couple who conceived me when my mother was 45. My father was a General in the Italian army, even if he received the title when he was a pensioner. A man of very few words, he was obsessed with order. Of him — he passed away a few years ago — I remember very few things, all of which are bad. We actually lived independent lives, and in the rare moments in which we were together, we used to ignore each other. He wanted me to become a medical doctor, like his father, and

* Sandro's real name has been changed to protect the privacy of the contributor.

~ 99 ~

when I communicated to him my intention to study at the conservatorium, he said: 'I don't know what is in your mind, but you are certainly not my son. You cannot be my son.'

He was accustomed to keeping order, even in the cupboard where Mum kept pasta and cookies. Believe it or not, he used to seal the open boxes of biscuits with sticky tape. I never saw him giving a kiss or a caress to my mother, and I am still bewildered as to how they could have had a sexual life together. They hated each other.

Arianna, my wife, has always been a very beautiful woman. I met her when I started my first year at the conservatorium. She was 18, and working as a waitress at the cafeteria opposite the main entrance of the conservatorium. I was 20, and I suffered from any remarks that other guys would make about her. I was incredibly jealous, even though we were not together. I spent months thinking about how I could approach her without being refused. I was shy and insecure, but one day I put a written request in her hand asking her out for dinner. To my great surprise, she did not say no. Just two years later we were husband and wife, much too young.

She continued with her job for a while. I played in piano bars here and there and the money was rather good. I still don't understand how I was able to do that job, with my shyness and all the rest. People liked my voice. I was good at performing Elton John songs. They really liked that.

When I finished my studies, I immediately won a piano competition, which gave me access to some good circles. I gave quite a number of concerts. However, what worked in the piano bars did not work in big auditoriums, and any time I had to play in concert was a calvary. The tension was so much that Arianna soon stopped following me to different cities. She could not cope with my tension and my violent reactions to everything.

A career under threat

I started drinking; I felt I could stand it better that way. But this remedy was not effective for very long. At the age of 30, I had my first admission to the hospital, and for a time my promising career as a pianist was close to a premature and ignoble end.

At that time, Arianna was just beginning a new job in a travel agency, something that she liked a lot. When out of the hospital, I promised Arianna my drinking would stop. She wanted me to give piano lessons and play in piano bars again, as this produced good money and was not perceived as distressing to me.

Although very humiliated by this perspective, and by my own behaviour in general, I tried to do it, and for a couple of months it more or less worked. For a very short time, we enjoyed some financial freedom and were on very good terms with each other. We bought a new kitchen. Then I wanted to get rid of the only concert that remained in my calendar from the year before. After a fierce argument with my wife, I convinced her to let me go. I was confident that I could manage it. The program involved Ravel, Stravinsky and Debussy, nothing too difficult for me since I knew the pieces in depth.

The night before the concert I could not sleep at all. By the morning, I was totally drunk. When Arianna called me around noon to wish me good luck, I could hardly pick up the phone. She then called the organisers to cancel the performance. I continued drinking until the arrival of my wife and her brother, to bring me home. That was the end of my career as a pianist. I never held another concert. Exactly eight months later, Arianna abandoned me. Every good intention had not worked and drinking was the only serious commitment that I had.

Whom to blame?

I went to the hospital again and afterwards I stayed at my mother's place for a while. I cannot remember precisely how many days I spent doing absolutely nothing, but certainly a good number. Mum was crying all the time, blaming herself for marrying my father and not giving me the warmth and serenity that is needed for raising children in the proper way.

After two months of that torture, I convinced my mother to let me go back to my apartment. Once home, I found a letter from Arianna informing me about a number of her recent decisions, including seeing someone else, whom she called a 'real man for a change'.

I was an alcoholic, with no job, and no one to talk to. A few days later, I decided that it was time to put into operation what I had been thinking for months, and what I considered the only plausible way to exit that unbearable situation. I had already prepared everything. What was missing was simply the when.

I had great difficulty in falling asleep at night. I could hardly put together 2 hours of sleep, with no naps during the day. I was tense and very, very, irritable, yelling at mum if she tried to ask me how I was. One night, around 2 a.m., I thought it was the moment. I dressed myself, and I drove up to the place where I knew Arianna was living with her new man. Their condominium had a private parking area. To access it, it was as easy as removing a little plastic covered chain. I was going to gas myself, over there.

It took me only 5 minutes to set up the procedure: the hose, the connection to the pipe, the sticky-tape, switching on the engine. From where I parked, I could see one of the windows of Arianna's apartment. I wanted her to see my corpse, the next day.

I had a bottle of cognac with me, and I immediately put down a big sip. Then I started writing my final letter. I wanted to address it to Arianna and to my Mum, but was not sure about the right order, maybe Mum and then Arianna. And why not to my father? I had so much to tell him, it really did not matter if he couldn't read it anymore. I finally started with 'To Whom It May Concern'. Most of the letter was for Arianna. I missed her unbearably, but I was aware that I could not render anyone happy, given my life. Her decision to go was damn right; I probably hated her because of this. She was always right, I was always wrong. She had always been better than me: more reliable, more serene, more beautiful and clean, inside and outside. She was strong enough to take care of two people, herself and me: her husband, a much more delicate and weak individual. She was for a long time able to tolerate my mood swings, my uncontrollable tension, and my being drunk anytime I shouldn't be. She even believed my promises fabricated out of alcohol. She let me think that I could be better that what I was. She was wonderful too much for me.

My final letter had to be comprehensive and detailed, I had to get rid of all my complaints against the world. Shamelessly, I truly wanted to leave an imprint on my survivors, Arianna and Mum, whose life — for sure — would not have been the same anymore, after my departure. Maybe the gas poisoning obliged me to cut the letter shorter than what I wanted (how long would it have lasted? — 10, 15, perhaps 20 minutes?). At some point, I felt my writing was fading away and I struggled to put my signature to it. Then, evidently, I fell unconscious.

I still have a copy of that letter. My mother gave it to me. It is just a photocopy, and I am not sure who possesses the original; mum, the police, or who knows whom. I only know that the content of that script still scares me. I find it difficult to recognise myself, today, in those lines. The accusations, the anger, the threats, everything it contains. Is too much, it is excessive. I wonder how I can still stand the gaze of my mother. I feel very full of shame for all of it.

Arianna did not want to see me anymore. I know for sure that she was given a copy of the letter, but instead of confronting me, she preferred to write back, after a while. Honestly, I don't even remember what she wrote to me. Probably she didn't say anything in particular. She was certainly happy that I was alive and that my attempt failed, with best wishes for my 'new' life. Well, it really is another life, but I have yet to say what happened to me that kept me in this world.

Another life, another chance

I survived for two main reasons. First, I tried to gas myself in a one-year-old car with a very good catalytic converter. Second, someone from the condominium going fishing early in the morning called the police. And, third, the subsequent hospital experience had a very salutary effect.

They brought me to the hospital where I stayed for three weeks, initially in the intensive care unit followed by five days in the psychiatric ward. I had been in hospital before for my drinking habits, but never in the psychiatric department. It was an appalling experience. I am not saying that I am normal and that I should not have been sent there (you have to be insane to become an alcoholic), but I surely didn't feel I was like 'them'. I wanted to get out of that frightening place as soon as possible. From this point of view, it was a very therapeutic experience; it really gave me the starting point, for my new life in the world of normalcy. However, as I said, this was not due to the treatment. I wonder how it is possible to recover from anything inside there. You are locked in there with a good number of very crazy people. They scream, they threaten you, they fight with each other or with the nurses. They cry all day. I was really terrified. I was sharing the same room with a young fellow who would say nothing but stare at me all the time. I could never sleep because I was in a state of panic, despite the many pills I was receiving. I had reduced myself to sleeping only at the time of visits and during meals, these were the less dangerous moments.

I believe I was discharged, not because of my clinical improvement, but because there were probably more severe cases to admit. Whatever the reason, I felt so relieved that my mother's house seemed like a real haven to me (and I had never felt at home there before!).

Today, I don't think anymore of those times. I re-married a year ago, and my new wife is seven months pregnant. I work in an insurance company, and I have more money that I ever felt possible in my previous life. However, I do not touch a piano anymore. I am too scared. Maybe one day my fingers will run over the black and white of a keyboard, but surely not in the near future. My memories are still too bad to see myself sitting in front of a piano. I am not listening to classical music either, which I once adored. Even, musical pauses over the phone scare me: I can't stand listening to *Für Elise* from Beethoven, and I often drop the line.

I sold my piano and tried to give the money that I obtained to my mother, but she refused. It was a gift for me, and gifts should never be returned. I then bought some furniture for my new apartment, particularly for the room designed for Alex, the baby whose arrival we are expecting in two months.

Diego, believe it or not, I still own my car, 'that' car. I am very resistant to selling it. It saved my life, and I am now very grateful for this. Very, very much so.

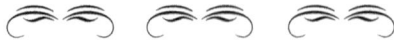

DIEGO'S COMMENTS ON SANDRO'S STORY

This story is both predictable and poignant. It is predictable because the break-up of a relationship is all too frequently a spur to suicidal behaviour, especially in males. Separation and loss often find them unprepared, be they young or old. Compared to women, men lack the capacity to cope with a lonely life, a life where they are often separated from their children and living in financial constraints. Sometimes even the little things of daily life, the cooking, the cleaning, may become an unbearable burden.

Australian statistics provide chilling evidence that separation from an intimate is the most frequent life event in the year preceding suicide. To understand this sad fact, we need to keep the following in mind. Men are not protected by the network of social relationships that characterises the female world. Men are mostly alone; and even if they have a few good mates, they talk very little with them, and certainly not about those things that are torturing their hearts. Thus, their instinct is to 'isolate': they don't like to show vulnerabilities or defeats. Research shows that men often think that their peers would not understand their private suffering; and that, if confessed, this could make them seem weak — a 'loser'. They already feel ashamed and their self-esteem has taken a battering.

Clearly, society's perception of masculinity — and, indeed, sex roles in general — is a major factor in this system of beliefs. Reduced or lost contact with children (with the added sting, sometimes, of an domestic violence order) adds to the total burden, and further contributes to the sense of emptiness in a life already felt as lacking basic meaning. Financial difficulties may represent the last straw.

Sandro does not resist the separation; does not argue with his wife; and does not behave violently. However, his aggression is evident in his plan of killing himself in full view of the windows of his estranged wife, now living with a new partner, a 'real man'. The pianist hopes that his wife will, the next day, see his dead body, and in this way finally realise how important she was to him. And also — I stress — she would have felt guilty, and responsible for causing his suicide.

So, in his vengeful fantasy, his being found dead by the occupants of that unit, the product of a new idyllic relationship, would have seriously undermined the happiness of that couple, overshadowing forever their expectations of serenity and fulfilment. Early psychoanalysts like Freud and Menninger interpreted suicide as a 'missed homicide', an act in which the subject, instead of suppressing the life of the 'other', re-directed their aggression towards the 'self. As it applies to this story, it seems to me that there is little doubt that Sandro wanted to kill the newly constituted couple.

'The Missed Concert' is also a story of waste because there were many opportunities to intervene to unlink the chain of events that ultimately led to the serious suicide attempt of its protagonist.

Sandro is a talented man, sensitive, reserved and insecure. Yes, he is confident enough to play and sing in piano bars; however, for formal and demanding events like concerts — something that he reveres — his anxiety grows in leaps and bounds, easily transformed into panic. As often happens to control tension, the pianist calls alcohol to his aid. But this is the worst self-therapy, and it rapidly fails. At the beginning, as do all new alcoholics, he genuinely believes that he can overcome his dependence at any time. He promises his wife he will stop drinking, but the promises are frequent and unkept, and the distance with his wife increases with each failure. Finally, the planned concert represents not only his last career opportunity, but also his last hope for a life change. Our pianist knows it well: that is why anxiety devours him. He will eventually drown all his uncertainties and hesitations in a sea of alcohol, and also sink his marriage.

Now, aware that his world is falling apart, he will never be able to cancel the negative image of himself that his father had underlined so many times, and he is sure that his wife will leave him. In sum, he feels that he is failing in all fronts, and the idea of suicide start growing quite rapidly in him. He writes that he has considered suicide for long time; he is only uncertain about the 'when'.

Today, Sandro is no longer a pianist; he has sold his instrument and does not even consider putting his fingers to a keyboard — it is still too disturbing. But he has re-balanced his life, and learnt from his near-fatal experience. Now his little son Alex represents his future, and, since he has been granted a second chance, he is striving to be a different type of father from his own father — less obsessed with ambition and orderliness, much more humane and sensitive.

EIGHT

≈ ≈

Country Living

*Fabrizio's Story**

*D*ear Diego,
It is not difficult to tell my story. I just fear it may be a bit boring.

My name is Fabrizio and I am now 55 years old and live with my 83-year-old mother. Overall, she is in better health than me. My health conditions have improved anyway. I suffer from bipolar disorder diagnosed at the age of 22. Maybe even before that time I was not completely normal. I have always been a bit 'up'. My friends wanted me to be always with them, because they liked my company. I was always kidding and making jokes. I loved to surprise the others.

When we lived in the Italian countryside with my dad and uncle, we also had a couple of horses and I had great fun with them. I used to ride without a saddle and was able to stand up over Tobia, my uncle's horse. The scar that I have under the chin was made by him, from when he kicked me when I was 15. They told me the surgeon worked more than five hours to repair my face and make it presentable again. But at the time I didn't care too much. On the contrary, I thought that the scar was something that would gain me the respect of my peers.

---

* Fabrizio's real name has been changed to protect the privacy of the contributor.

I was hard to manage in those days. I remember once, with two friends of mine, we were blowing paper bullets with a pin on the top towards the testicles of one of the bulls that we had. The bull became furious and broke the door of its box in the stable, running all around. My mother and my uncle had to call the firemen and the veterinary doctor to calm it down and bring it back to the stable. I hid in the hayloft with my friends. The bull took several hours to recover, and when my father came back home, he beat me with his trouser belt. The next day I could not attend school because I could not sit. From that moment on I was not allowed to bring any friends home.

My father was a policeman. He worked in the Traffic Department. My uncle, his brother, managed the farm. My grandfather had left us that property. We were not rich, but not poor either. At home we had everything we needed. My father had never had a great relationship with his father, my grandfather. That is why he did something very different from him. He said that to be a farmer was a dirty job. He didn't want to have anything to do with cattle, nor did he want to kill animals, particularly pigs. We had many of them, and it was my uncle who took care of everything. However, my father loved salami and sausages. My uncle never stopped reminding him, while eating salami, that this delicious food was the product of his 'dirty' work. Had my father been an honourable man, he would have avoided eating them. I think that my father was angry about the teasing, but I know that he was willing to forgive my uncle anyway.

My uncle was five years older than my father, but 20 cm shorter. However, he was as strong as two men. He was a very quiet person; I never saw him with any women. If someone said something about this, he replied that he was forced to sacrifice his life in order to run the farm, or else everything could have turned out badly. What is true is that he had one of those characters that render problematic any contact with other human beings. He was quite talkative with his animals, but never with people. I have a clear memory of him always accompanied by a tiny dog, a black and white cross, which he called 'Bone'. This little animal really stuck by his side. I never saw my uncle caressing that dog, which followed him everywhere, even on the top of Tobia when my uncle rode, or drove the tractor.

Strangely, he showed some affection for a cat, a big wandering male, unapproachable by all but my uncle. 'Moustache' was its name. Actually, it was surprising to see a nearly wild animal so docile and at ease under the huge and rough hands of my uncle. Maybe they were two good examples of wildness, and that's why they went well together.

He had no words with my mother either. Sometimes my uncle said 'Good-day' to her; most of the time, nothing. With my father he would only discuss money. However, I believe that he had a particular eye for me. He was the one who taught me to ride. When Tobia ruined my chin, there was a violent argument in the family. When I came home from the hospital, I heard my father saying to my mother that his brother had said 'strange things' that he didn't like at all. I believe that those strange things became a reality years later. I was studying at the home of a friend — I can remember it as though it was yesterday — and Dad rang to call me back home. Something serious had happened to my uncle.

I was in the second year of my university course of engineering. I wanted to build bridges one day. I immediately realised that something serious could only mean one thing: that my uncle had died. And this was, in fact, the case.

At the age of 55, right on the day of his birthday, my uncle had decided to forever leave his solitary and silent life, together with his 'dirty' job, and gunned himself down with his double-barrel. It was 11 a.m., and he did it in his bedroom. When my father rang me, they had already taken away his body and cleaned his room.

My mother said later that she had suspected something when she saw him coming home at that unusual time of the day. They were harvesting wheat during that time, and there was a lot to do. It seems also that my uncle had, incredibly, requested her to prepare something special for dinner: 'You are 55 only once,' he added, as if to justify his unexpected request. 'How special? Mum replied. 'This is up to you', he dryly said.

In the city

After my uncle's death, my mother did not want to live in the countryside anymore. On the other hand, there was nobody to deal with the farm. Consequently, we decided to live in the city, where I was already attending the university. A few months later, our farm was sold out. With that money we bought an apartment where my mother and I still live.

Once in the new place, I fell ill for the first time. Quite clearly, my uncle's suicide shocked me, even if I have no recollection of having spent too much time thinking about it. I would not consider myself as cynical, but I often had the impression that my uncle was too strange a personality to have lived happily in this world. He had a hard life without any friend or woman.

At that time, I was madly in love with Luisa. She was a girl who was studying mathematics and had the sweetest eyes that I had ever seen. I had noticed her in the university Mensa, and since then I couldn't stop thinking about her. Unfortunately, after a few months of great love together, Luisa told me that I was not the man she was looking for, that she did not love me any more, and that I had to look for another woman. I could not stop thinking about Luisa. I could not sleep or be involved in anything constructive or positive. I stopped studying completely. But at some point it was clear that I was out of order. I started thinking that I loved everybody and that everybody loved me. I started kissing people on the street, and I even thought that my uncle was protecting me and also encouraging me in that behaviour from heaven. Someone reacted to my effusions and slapped me.

I ended up in a psychiatric ward, taken there by force. I stayed there for approximately 40 days. They initially said that I suffered from schizophrenia, that I was talking to Jesus Christ, and that I was hearing voices that existed only inside my head. Then they changed their minds. After a few other admissions, I was transformed into a 'bipolar'. Strangely enough, medications remained the same. I was not too compliant — anytime I felt better, I regularly stopped taking them.

I wanted to study, to graduate, and to build my bridges. Under medication you cannot study. Your brain doesn't work properly, you feel stoned. Your head is heavy, your reactions are slow, your thoughts too. This was exactly the opposite of when I was OK, before the illness, when my brain was fast and everything was easy for me. I walked like a robot, my legs felt like two pieces of wood. If I tried to study, my eyes began to burn, and my vision blurred.

Before my 'bipolarity' I had all my examinations done in due time, with excellent marks. Then, in over four to five years I had successfully completed only two exams. In sum, I felt that I could not make it any more. I also had terrible periods of black depression. This is the worst thing that can happen to you. It is much better hearing voices than feeling down in that way. You cannot understand what depression is like if you haven't experienced it. The world has no more colours, nothing interests you, and nobody attracts you. There is no life in things. There is no need to eat, no desire to wash yourself. Just dark night.

Meanwhile my father had died from myocardial infarction. He left my mother with a small pension and a mentally ill child. I imagine that for my mother it must have been an incredibly difficult period. In a few years she had to cope with the discovery of the body of my uncle, her widowhood, and my psychiatric condition. But she has an iron will, that lady. I always thought that. On the other hand, her life with my father would not have been too easy. Born in the city centre, she was convinced by him to live in the countryside, with more contact with my uncle (whatever the meaning of contact was with him) than with my father. She adapted well to everything, poor woman, and even if she looked like a little bird, small as she was, she has always demonstrated the strength of a giant. And I have greatly contributed to rendering her life more and more difficult.

If only

It was after a hospital admission for an episode of depression, the fourth or fifth from the beginning of my illness, I believe, that I had started thinking about committing suicide. Realising that my life could not return to normal, I knew I would never ever become an engineer. I never confessed these feelings to my mother, but I talked about it with some doctors. They told me that thinking about suicide is absolutely usual when you are depressed. It is the condition that leads you in this direction.

In hospital, during a previous admission, I had met a girl whom I liked very much. It was not like being with Luisa, but at least this person seemed truly and constantly interested in me. We made a number of plans for our future. We also fantasised about living together one day. When I said something about Katia to my mother, she strongly discouraged me. She didn't think that my situation would allow any investment in another person. I had to wait until my full recovery. If only it could have happened ...

Katia was quite secretive about herself. Once out from the hospital, we were to meet on very few occasions. We made love during one of those meetings. Then, one day, I rang her doorbell but nobody replied. Only some months later, on the occasion of that fourth or fifth admission for a depressive episode, I learnt that Katia had hanged herself. I still don't know how much this event shocked me. I think it had enormous significance for my subsequent behaviour.

Psychiatrists discharged me because I looked much improved; at least this was the appearance. Once at home, I remember that my mother started cooking and I went straight to her bedroom, knowing that in the bedside table my father's police revolver was still there. For some reason, this had not been returned to police authorities. It was unloaded, but I knew were to find the bullets. I put the pistol under my pillow and joined my mother in the kitchen. My mind was totally concentrated on my project: I would wait until Mum have started washing dishes and I would go downstairs to the cellar. There, in a certain cupboard, I would find the bullets, and there I would do it. I didn't want my mother to clean away new blood from her house.

What sort of book?

I tried to eat as much as I could so my mother did not become suspicious. Despite my apparent appetite, she said that I didn't look very well and it would be better for me to stay in hospital a bit longer. I remember very clearly her words because she had to repeat them hundreds of time. After the meal, I went down to the cellar with the pretext of picking up some old books. 'What sort of book are you looking for?' asked Mum. Expecting a similar enquiry, I was ready to provide an answer: 'Moby Dick. In hospital they told me that it is a great book, but when I read it I simply thought that it was OK. That is why I want to re-read it'.

I think my heart was beating fast. Rather strangely, while my head was in complete turmoil, my movements were correct and coordinated. I went to my bedroom to get the revolver from under the pillow. I put it in my pocket and went down the stairs. No, I did not feel normal at all. But for how long had I not felt normal anymore?

I immediately found the cartridges. I had never previously loaded my father's revolver, but I had seen him unloading it so many times. I loaded the firearm without any difficulty, I pushed the safety-bolt, and I sat on the floor, my legs crossed.

I put my left hand over my chest searching for the point in which the heart was beating stronger. With the barrel I pushed aside my left fingers and applied the revolver. I felt in a hurry: my mother might have imagined everything and distracted me from my proposal. I had to act rapidly. I said to myself that there was nothing to re-think and the decision was well taken.

I closed my eyes and pulled the trigger.

I was waiting for a burning pain. Nothing. Nothing happened. Actually, something had happened for sure, but not in the way I was expecting. I felt some painful sensation, but quite light and not comparable to what I was prepared to face. Maybe I was in the process of dying or already dead and this was just the beginning of the afterlife. I felt that I could not open my eyes. When I finally succeeded, the first thing I saw was the eyes, full of terror and tears, of my mother.

Still alive

I was still alive, my heart still beating. Only my breathing was a bit different. I had missed my target! I was in the surgical department, then in the psychiatric ward. In two months I was back home. That time I felt much better. And happy to be alive, incredibly. I honestly don't know the reason for this shift in thinking. Why did I change my mind so dramatically? Destiny had opposed my attempt: I had to take into account this factor. Having been so close to death had in some way regenerated my life, evidently. I can't find the right explanation, even if I asked it of myself a million times. Sometimes I have the feeling that I have cancelled a kind of responsibility.

I have been admitted to the hospital on several occasions since, but my crises were somehow lighter and less intense.

Furthermore, I had the impression that doctors treated me in a very different way, much more carefully than before. It is 10 years now since I have been taking lithium. I also have an injection every month. It is eight years since my last admission. My health is much better than before. Sadly, Diego, I never worked, I never became an engineer, and my bridges have remained in my fantasy. However, I read a lot and I enjoy doing it. I spend many hours on the Internet, which is really incredible stuff. I do not think about killing myself anymore.

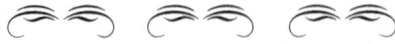

DIEGO'S COMMENTS ON FABRIZIO'S STORY

The sad legacy of mental disorders is once again in evidence in this extraordinary tale, with its protagonist suffering from a major disorder, probably a bipolar disorder, though hearing voices is not really typical of this picture. It is also unclear why this man was given an injection every month of a long-acting neuroleptic (a drug to control psychotic experiences). However, sometimes doctors continue with the same prescriptions just because patients are doing OK, even if the medications given do not really correlate with the diagnosis. And, of course, patients do not always match textbook descriptions; anyway, in this case all ended well.

Two tragic events paved the way to the suicidal behaviour of the protagonist of this story, reminding us of the role of this type of knowledge in the determinism of a suicidal act. The first involved Fabrizio's uncle, a sort of 'half-man, half-animal'; in any case, a rather wild creature, certainly not adept in human interactions, but probably quite fond of our protagonist. The space that this uncle is given in the story indicates his importance for Fabrizio, even if the latter says that at the time of his uncle's death he did not think too much about that terrible event. However, perhaps not by chance, Fabrizio also tried to use a firearm to kill himself, as did his uncle.

The suicide of Katia is an obvious and powerful trigger for Fabrizio's suicide attempt. He was very taken with her; even accepting her disappearing for months at a time (psychiatric patients are incredibly tolerant of each other), and this girl probably represented an opportunity for change in his life after its disillusions (the psychiatric disease, his shattered career as bridge designer, the end of his love story with Luisa, and so on). Katia gave him the sensation that spreading his wings was still possible.

As Fabrizio recounts, the tragic death of Katia is deeply shocking and destined to have 'enormous significance' on his subsequent behaviour. After all, a suicide is also a rejection of the other/s, and among the million thoughts and attempts to find a plausible explanation, the protagonist has probably felt this, especially in light of the many projects they fantasised together.

Admitted to a psychiatric ward following a new episode of depression, our protagonist is discharged, looking 'much improved'. And immediately his suicidal plan becomes operational. I have heard on so many occasions of a similar circumstance: depressed patients present with a marked amelioration in their clinical picture and this — together with the perennial pressure on hospital beds — justifies their release from the ward. While we cannot blame doctors for this, experience (and a lot of literature) teaches us that the post-discharge period represents a very delicate balance with regard to the suicide risk. In fact, paradoxically, severe depressive symptomatology may actually be 'protective' for patients, by inhibiting dangerous initiatives. Once the burden of depression is somewhat lifted — for example, at the beginning of antidepressant treatment — and patients become less 'inhibited' and more mobile and active, they may also be more inclined to transform their depressive thoughts into action. Suicide then becomes possible.

This seems to have been the case for our protagonist. Once at home, he puts in action his deadly plan. The availability of a pistol facilitates it. That the suicide of his uncle is on his mind at the time of the attempt is evident by the reference to his mother, years before forced to clean the mess in the room of her brother-in-law; he will avoid causing her the same type of problem.

He pulls the trigger. Then comes a moment when he is unable to understand if he is already dead or still alive. When he realises that he is destined to continue living, he is happy to be alive. He feels 'regenerated'.

Many years later, our protagonist seems to have completely eradicated all suicidal ideation from his thoughts. He is grateful for the second chance granted to him. Miracles do happen.

⤢ ⤡

NINE

A Busy Husband

Lucia's Story *

*D*ear Diego,

I have so much to be thankful for and welcome the opportunity to share my experience with others.

I am 47 years old and I live in Milan. I have two children; both of them are independent and are doing well. Both are very reliable people. My husband is 53 and he directs a museum of arts. He is also involved in politics and is very involved with both commitments. I was a teacher for more that 20 years. I have a brother, Pietro, who is much younger than me. We have never had a great relationship. He never married. He takes care of many acres that my father left us and lives with my mother, who will be 70 soon.

It was my brother who discovered the body of our father, more than 20 years ago. My father hanged himself in the garage of our old house. He had suffered with bipolar disorder for his entire life. In the period immediately prior to his death, he thought that he had brought our family to ruin, that in a short time there would be no more bread on our table, and that agriculture was the worst occupation to choose in the world.

Nobody could change his mind. Following electroconvulsive therapy sessions, he looked better and was discharged from the hospital. Two days later he killed himself.

* Lucia's real name has been changed to protect the privacy of the contributor.

I remember that it was around 5 o'clock in the evening on a late September day. It had rained for nearly all the day, that Thursday. My brother insisted we go for a bike ride but my mother didn't approve. 'It will rain again,' she said. Pietro replied that he needed to stretch a bit before it was dark and time for dinner. I said nothing, as I was sure that he wouldn't listen to me. He never listened to me. He saw me as the boring sister, and one mother for him was more than enough. While going to grab his bike, he saw the corpse.

I shall never forget his face when he came back to tell us what he had seen. That fact changed his life forever, I believe. It changed the lives of all of us forever. My mother has not been the same since. After so many years, Pietro still has anger inside him, and I am not at all surprised that he hasn't found a partner. Even if he is only 39, I know that he will never change for the better. And Mum? She is a disaster. Her only social activity, since then, is to go to the church. Nothing else.

A way out?

I felt that I couldn't live in that house anymore. So, at 24 I got married. At the beginning, I thought that I loved my husband Antonio. He was already much taken by his work, but he was very polite and respectful (something unusual in the country-side) and with a cultured background that I admired very much. Almost immediately I had two children, one after the other. Soon I realised that it was not real love: he was looking for a family, possibly by marrying a wealthy women, and I was trying to escape from home. Sex was never an issue in our marriage, in the sense that it happened very seldom but nobody complained about that. Raising my kids and teaching at the local secondary school was all that I've done, for many, many years.

Antonio became successful in his profession very early on. When he started to direct the museum he was not yet 35. After that, it was just work, work and work again. I am still wondering if he has ever had other affairs with anyone else. How could a man live without sex?

Three years ago I jumped from the third floor of my city flat. Why and how I survived God only knows. Incredibly, it happened. I have thought about that day many times, but I have no recollection of any particular feeling, no premonitory signs. Yes, I was particularly tired from my school teaching, but I had felt the same way on many other occasions. I had the sensation of a never-ending anxiety, which I had been living with for a long time.

That day — very hot and humid — my husband wanted me to accompany him to the official opening of a new pavilion at the museum. I had to assume the role of the good wife, as required by the circumstances. I have played that part hundreds of time before and always with the same lack of enthusiasm you feel when you are very sleepy but you still have to brush your teeth prior to going to bed. Very boring then, but I knew that I had to do it. It was in our non-spoken agreement.

That morning my husband was particularly tense. He has always been a nervous person. On that occasion it was the delayed arrival of the Mayor that troubled him. His participation was in doubt, since he had to arrive from a previous commitment in a faraway city. The ceremony was fixed for noon. My husband had been in contact with the Mayor's secretary by phone since early in the morning.

We live in the countryside, then as well as now. Antonio decided to buy a flat in the city to allow our children to be closer to university and to friends. He used to sleep there quite often, the museum being in walking distance. For the inauguration he suggested that we sleep there, but I hated that place, so impersonal and cold. I said that there was enough time to reach the museum from our country house without rushing too much.

On the road to the opening, my husband decided that he had to change his shirt, which was wet from sweating so much. In the city, at the entrance to the building, I asked him if I could wait for him in the car. I felt tense and disappointed by the unexpected stop. 'Come up', he said, 'It will only be a matter of a minute, it's too hot to wait in the car'. OK, then. I entered the building with him. I never used the lift. He did, I climbed the stairs. I felt my anxiety growing step by step.

In the flat, he made a few phone calls, probably checking about the Mayor. I felt too nervous to sit. I remember that I tried to control my tension by breathing deeply. Finally, he changed his damn shirt and we went down.

When he turned the key to start the engine, I asked him to wait because I needed the toilet. 'Are you nuts? We'll be late!' He looked at me as if I had disobeyed an order of vital importance. 'Why didn't you use the toilet when we were upstairs? One of these days we have to talk seriously, the two of us. We need to clarify something.' He was right, we had to clarify a lot of things, I thought.

I climbed the stairs again. It was suffocating inside there. My head was so heavy and my legs grew increasingly weaker. I didn't need to use the toilet. It was not clear what brought me up there. I needed more air. I opened the door of the balcony and the sun nearly pushed me back. I didn't look down, I didn't hesitate — I just closed my eyes and I jumped. In the few seconds of the fall, I thought that I was going to put an end to everything that was horrible and senseless. I was going to free myself, forever.

I would like to say more about it, but I can't really add too much. It was something that 'happened' to me quite suddenly. I had never seriously thought to commit suicide before. I could say that even that day I didn't previously think to kill myself ... It was a kind of sudden decision, something that became clear to me at the very last moment.

A new beginning

Anyway, landing on the cement was incredibly painful. I didn't lose consciousness. I heard the voices around me, someone was screaming. Curiously, my husband arrived after the ambulance (the balcony was on the other side of the entrance to the building, where we parked). My first worry was to verify if I could move my legs and arms, and yes, I could. There was no blood around me, and I remember people saying: 'Don't touch her, don't move her, wait for the ambulance'. I heard other questions such as: 'Can you understand? Can you answer?' but more of: 'Be calm, don't worry, it's OK'. Actually, it was they who were agitated, not me.

I think that I must have lost consciousness in the ambulance. I remained in the hospital for two months with fractures everywhere. Afterwards, I needed further surgery for both my legs and was transported to a more specialised hospital in a different city. This meant nearly six months in all. Doctors were very concerned that I might try to kill myself again and, as a result, they put me in rooms on the first floor only. They also gave me antidepressant and sedative medication, I believe. I found it very difficult to sleep, as well as to maintain a comfortable posture when awake.

My life has changed a lot now. I feel my children are very close to me, as are both my mother and brother. My mother, in particular, is different towards me. It seems that she has a new sense in life now; after so many years, we can talk to each other again. This is very rewarding for me now.

My husband's behaviour has been impeccable. He did a lot for me. He found the best doctors, the best assistance, and was very efficient, indeed. He still says to others that he doesn't understand the reasons behind my act. I hope that, privately, he may know something more. Honestly, I am not sure about that. Our marriage is still there, but we know that it is finished forever. We live under the same roof, but we run separate and independent lives.

At the beginning, I hated the psychiatrist who was chosen for me. He was said to be the best, but I didn't want him. I felt that I didn't need a shrink and that it was too easy to label me as a psychiatric case. I thought that I simply needed more consideration and love, and not medicines and sessions with a psychiatrist. Was it really the best that my family could do for me?

Today I am very happy to have been 'assigned' to that man — to you, Diego. I have learned a lot about myself and others. I have meaning in my life that I didn't have before. I do not teach anymore. It cost me a lot reaching that decision, but I was sure that as a 'suicide attempter' I would not have any credibility. However, my life has never been as rewarding as it is today. I am fully committed to several volunteer activities, and I do a lot of physical exercise and I can walk perfectly, thank God. That was all necessary for my rehabilitation before; now it is essential for my wellbeing.

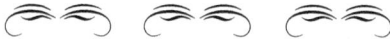

DIEGO'S COMMENTS ON LUCIA'S STORY

This story serves to highlight the patterns present in many suicides. Suicide, in itself 'unspeakable' in that there is no vocabulary to capture the experience or to allay its impact, can additionally cast a longer shadow. Such an act can bequeath a grim 'family script', a blueprint that can hold in thrall those left behind. First, the head of the family has taken his own life — deeply shocking in itself — and, next, he has done this in a way that means that his body will very likely be found by his family.

We are not party to the emotions of the protagonist's brother on the day that he discovered his father hanging in the garage; but certainly that experience changed forever the life of that young man and his entire family.

The father had bipolar disorder, a psychiatric condition characterised by volatile mood swings oscillating between depressive and manic states, with periods of wellbeing of variable duration. Severe bipolar disorder carries a high risk of suicide;[1] and in any case, when not pharmacologically controlled, it may heavily condition the life of affected individuals and those around them. The protagonist's story would suggest that her father was in the grip of a psychotic depression, and beset by delusional ideas of financial ruin. In short, a dangerous clinical picture. Unfortunately, no medical intervention was able to intercept that fatal trajectory.

It is obvious from her subsequent patterns that the suicide of her father severely affected the life of our protagonist and shaped her own suicidal behaviour. While superficially her suicide attempt looks sudden and impulsive, its origin is easily located in the adoption of the problem-solving strategy taught so tragically by her father.

There is a feeling of oppression and airlessness as the protagonist struggles to move out from the shadow of her father's legacy. First comes — that most common of mistakes — the early marriage, to escape from the suffocation of her family home; then the predictable consequences of a choice made in 'reaction' rather than freely chosen: lovelessness and duty, children and job plug the growing vacuum. On the surface an exemplary life, even enviable, but in reality a prison, a cage, and with less and less room to breathe. This spiral of circumstances and events is evident in her story, and culminates in her final bid for 'freedom'.

The way she climbs the stairs up to the third floor on that torrid day is described as if it was the logical epilogue of an entire life run without breathing. Her jump represented to her the 'only' possibility for freedom from the constraints shackling her to her daily life.

Her impulsive-seeming, unplanned suicidal act might be regarded as surprising in a mature adult, one who had been up until then so consistently reliable in her roles and behaviour. Surprisingly, many suicides, especially among such conventional people, involve little premeditation and the impulse is conceived only a few minutes before the act.[2] Though not disinhibited by alcohol, and lacking the desperate energy of the young, this middle-aged wife and mother of two, absolutely 'square', was suddenly overwhelmed by a surfeit of order and respectability and, burdened by everyone's needs, adopted her father's solution. A last cry for freedom.

I was fortunate to meet her again two years later. She now radiated happiness and vitality: her life had opened up. She was a devoted grandmother to her daughter's babies, had quit her teaching job, and had recently moved into a unit in the city. And she left her husband.

Notes

1   And sometimes of 'altruistic' homicide, in the belief that suppressing own proxies may avoid undue suffering to them.

2   The notorious 'party suicides' are a typical example of such cases; here individuals — in the absence of any obvious concerns — participate in a social event, and after a few drinks and probably a last-minute disappointment, impulsively decide, for example, to jump from the balcony.

≈ ≈

TEN

Afternoons on the Verandah

Umberto's Story

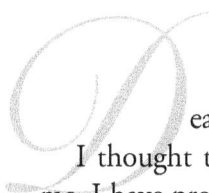

*D*ear Diego,

I thought that suicide was the only possible solution for me. I have prostate cancer, and I don't know how long I shall survive. I know for sure that at some point in time my situation seemed unbearable to me and that a quick exit looked like the most intelligent thing to do. I have been in a wheelchair for more than a year. I have a personal assistant for most of the day. Bathing my body and changing my clothes are distressing and painful procedures. My prostate cancer has produced metastases that have deeply altered my vertebra, particularly the lumbar ones, and consequently I cannot stand up any more. For more than three years I have been fighting this 'Calvary'. Today I would not make the same decision, but a year ago I felt quite different and the entire situation, as I said, looked unbearable to me.

This is what happened …

I live alone. My wife died 15 years ago from breast cancer. We had four children, all of them adorable, but completely absorbed in their own lives. My two sons live in the United States: one is a surgeon in a New York hospital and the other works on Wall Street. They each have two children. They are both successful and well.

My daughters live around here. They are very nice people. The youngest was married 18 months ago. They have always been very close to me and I cannot complain about anything. This is life; it is perfectly acceptable that everybody may live the way he or she chooses. Even if I have cancer, I don't want my daughters to sacrifice their lives to remain close to me. I don't need any more money than I have: I can pay for help, but I prefer to be alone during the night. I can manage it quite easily.

I still have some friends. One, in particular, is even more unfortunate than me. On a highway, a few years ago, a truck struck his car, killing his wife instantly and leaving him crippled and disfigured. It took him almost a year to recover from some of his injuries. Yes, he is alive, but he is a mess. I visited him several times in hospital, even after I was diagnosed with cancer. I have always liked to spend time with him. We felt like two shipwrecked men. We both survived our wives, we both had big physical problems; maybe his are bigger than mine. When we were together, we didn't say anything special. Probably it was more silence than talking, but we did not feel pressure to say something. We just enjoyed being in each other's company. We spent many afternoons at his place, particularly, on his verandah. Built at the beginning of the 20th century, his home is a three-storey building on the outskirts of the city. He likes to host me on the verandah. That space was originally a terrace on the first floor, but it was enclosed with glass, probably when his home was originally built, and the iron structure that supported the glass is in a nice Liberty style, without too many cavils. I believe that the remaining part of the house — large indeed — was too full of memories to enjoy it pleasantly.

Thus we silently agreed that the verandah was the right place to sit. There is fine furniture in bamboo and rattan, with the top of the tea-table and the cushioning of the chairs painted in floral motifs. He had placed a sheet of glass on the table to protect its surface. He had also put pillows everywhere, which surely gave me comfort. Afterwards, I simply positioned my wheelchair in the room. Tommaso, my unfortunate friend, had installed the facility for wheelchairs in his stairwell up to the second floor, and this was good for him and for me too. Evidently, he decided to renounce his third floor where, he told me, he put most of his wife's stuff.

From the verandah
On the verandah there were four lemon trees in beautiful handmade terracotta pots. After Tommaso's wife's death, only a few other plants (succulents) had survived, a bit like the two of us. And, like us, they looked hesitant about their future. From the verandah you could see the cupolas of the St Giustine cathedral, where I have never been in my entire life (I have always been a kind of priest-eater). But it was in that direction we both turned our eyes during our long silent periods, as that was the only point from which something unexpected could happen — who knows, perhaps something vaguely useful to us?

Actually, I cannot say what Tommaso was looking at: he had lost his right eye in the accident, and from the other he was left very short-sighted. Refusing a prosthesis or bandage, he wore black glasses that were probably capable of annihilating the sighting capacity of a hawk. Tommaso apparently didn't care about it. He had already seen enough in his life, he said once.

When I was with him, there, I was in charge of giving him his medication. These were scrupulously prepared by a nurse, who had been a friend of his wife for many years. Tommaso swallowed five or six different pills with a sip of water or orange juice. The only medicine that had attracted me from the beginning was the phenobarbital, a barbiturate — as the nurse explained — to avoid the danger of convulsions as a consequence of the terrible trauma that Tommaso had suffered.

Since I visited Tommaso on average every other day, I could take up to two phenobarbital pills per week away with me. In the beginning, I had strong feelings of guilt because of this (what would be the consequences for Tommaso?). Afterwards, I tried to remain in control by thinking that eventually I'd interrupt the dirty business as soon as the first signs of his discomfort were apparent. On the other hand, Tommaso seemed to be able to cope well even with half the dosage of his medication.

Thinking of Marilyn

I had heard and read a lot about barbiturates. You die, for sure, from an overdose of barbiturates. Marilyn Monroe taught the world about that. And she was the most beautiful and desirable woman on the planet. I mean, if she did it, I should have had very little to think about, given my being in a wheelchair, with the perspective of further suffering for the very short future left for me to live.

However, thinking of Marilyn increased my ambivalence. I was not totally sure that she had committed suicide. Actually, it was more probable that she was 'suicided' by someone else. Her doctors, for example, and particularly that famous Dr Greenson, the psychoanalyst who, apart from inviting her to dinner and taking her on family holidays, prescribed her large doses of barbiturates. What sort of psychoanalytic treatment was that? I had always been intrigued by the case of Ms Monroe, being — as had many millions of men throughout the world — an enchanted admirer of her astonishing femininity. Marilyn's case made me hate the category of psychiatrists/psychologists/psychoanalysts even more than priests. At least the latter approaches life a bit more moderately than the former. Is their 'science' any more grounded than that of astrologers and tarot readers?

When I was told that I would be confined to a wheelchair, I was also sent to a psychiatrist. For sure, that man was someone needing more help than me. I wonder why they do not check these people before sending them onto the battle-field. I can understand that to do that job you must be a bit 'strange'; otherwise you have no motivation for doing it. But there is a limit to everything!

Anyway, I stopped acquiring Tommaso's pills when I reached approximately 40 tablets. Based on my amateur knowledge, it was more than enough to die. I kept the pills inside a Limoges porcelain box where my wife once saved her jewels. Those pills were quite precious to me; they gave me a kind of additional power. I could reach my wife whenever I wanted, from now on. I was not a believer in the afterlife, and consequently I didn't really think about rejoining my wife. But the idea of putting my body to eternal rest, as it was for my wife, represented a growing seduction.

Why continue?

What was there to live for anyway? What should I expect from my future? I had no more responsibilities or tasks to attend to. All of my children were completely independent; certainly they didn't need me anymore. In addition, especially my daughters could have stopped visiting me. It was not a matter of doubting their love and devotion, but most of their visits were certainly the product of a moral imposition.

I don't know if I was a good father for them or not. I've always done my best for them, and my life has never gone beyond family and work. Anyway, I never doubted the love of my children. This was not the problem. Simply put, it was meaningless to continue. I didn't want to proceed further.

The anniversary of my wife's death would have occurred on a certain Sunday. That day fitted in with the scope available to me. The decision was made and my mind was finally very calm. My assistant went away every night at eight o'clock: I would act immediately after that. The following day, upon her return, she would have found my lifeless body. There was plenty of time to plan it carefully. And so I did.

I wrote a short letter to my children, one for all, in which I asked for an understanding response from them. They would have understood, I was sure.

Then I wrote a message to Tommaso. In his case I felt much less confident. I feared that I could easily influence his enormously difficult life, and very negatively too. I could not forgive myself for this. In my explanations to him, I wrote that, contrary to his case, my condition would have rapidly worsened anyway. More suffering, more medical visits, more interventions. More money spent, more assistance, more concern from my children. Better to end it as soon as possible: 'Meaningless to continue, Tommaso. That's why you have to excuse me, and don't even think to imitate me. Your dear friend, Umberto'.

These were, more or less, my final words to him, written after many hesitations over another important point: should I have mentioned to him about the stealing of his pills, and maybe thanked him for his involuntary but crucial help in providing the lethal weapon? No, the matter was too complicated and dangerous to be brought to his attention in that way. I admired and loved Tommaso, and I didn't want to create any further shock in addition to my departure. Better to skip the issue completely. Maybe one day he would have known that I died through an overdose of pills, but most probably the nature of the pills would have remained a forensic issue, and surely their origin a perennial mystery.

I found it very convincing, and I started to empty the content of the porcelain box onto the palm of my hand. I swallowed a few of them with a sip of cold milk that I used to drink every night before sleeping. I repeated the operation five or six times: Very easy. Since I was already in bed, I pulled the blanket up to cover my chin. I looked at my old travel clock, covered with bright vellum (those that you fold twice to put them back), and I noticed for the first time that its brand, 'Veglia', in Italian means also 'vigil'.

Twenty past eight. A bit early for going to bed maybe, but that evening was really a special evening. 'Goodnight, world. Better, goodbye', I said to myself.

I closed my eyes and joined my hands over my chest. I was really calm, much more than the many times in which I had tried to imagine that moment. The eternal sleep would arrive soon; I was very sure about that.

Despite my great confidence, I woke up three days later in an intensive care unit. My son Alex, the surgeon from New York, was passing by heading to Rome for a medical congress and had decided to make a surprise visit. At nine o'clock, after ringing unsuccessfully at my door and phoning with no reply, he had gone to his youngest sister and, with her keys, found me unconscious — but still alive — in my bedroom. A few minutes more, and perhaps his attempts would have been useless. That is what happened and that is why I am here to report my story.

Back to the verandah

It has been striking indeed, the coincidence between my attempt and Alex's arrival. I have no memory of similar visits from him. Perhaps he thought that, as I was dying from cancer, every possible occasion for being close to me should not be missed. The previous Christmas he could not come to visit me. Both his children had a bout of the flu, and I preferred not to insist. Certainly the coincidence between his arrival and my imminent departure is something unreal, nearly impossible to believe. It holds plenty of meaning for my subsequent life.

Actually, I felt very bad after the 'accident', even if my malaise was very different from the gloomy resignation that dictated my death project. For many days I felt very ashamed and mean. I thought that I had been a poor example to my children. I should have taught them about dignity and strength of character, even when life does not seem worth living.

As you know, Diego, as a psychiatrist with a normal face and behaviour, you helped me a lot on that occasion. You made me aware of my depression and how this pathology had influenced my suicide plans. You gave me a therapy that made me feel better very quickly. I wonder why other psychiatrists never suggested any drug for me.

At the beginning, Alex wanted to bring me to the United States because he did not trust the Italian doctors. But he is an Italian doctor, even if he is operating in America for more than 20 years and now has a big reputation. A meeting with the new psychiatrist convinced him to leave me here, under the care of the Italian doctor.

Now I am not too bad. Chemotherapy seems to be quite effective, at least it has stabilised my cancer. My oncologist says nothing, but smiles at me a bit more than before. I continue with my antidepressants; if this is the result, I am quite happy with it.

I have resumed my afternoons with Tommaso — on his verandah, as before, but we talk much more now. I can say that we really talk about everything. We talk about God, religion and the afterlife, but we also share our juvenile love stories. Even sex is a topic in our discussion now. We both deeply loved our wives, but we discovered that we also got up to some pranks years ago …

I'll die when God decides so. Evidently, he didn't want me to die last year, and I am grateful to Him for it. I learned a lot of new things about life and myself.

Dear Diego, I deeply thank all who have helped me, even though my words will never be enough to describe what I feel inside. Many thanks, anyway.

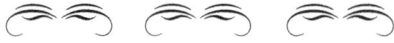

DIEGO'S COMMENTS ON UMBERTO'S STORY

In this tale, another Phoenix resurrects from the ashes of a much shaken life, a life irremediably compromised by cancer, one of our most powerful and dangerous enemies.

Umberto faces the prospect of only further suffering and worry — useless, he thinks — for the short time that remains to his life. Widowed, not religious (but spiritual, even if not a 'true believer'), well educated (note his comments on Marilyn Monroe and her doctor), Umberto sees no future for himself. Or, at least, not a liveable future. He is clearly without hope, and depressed.

I included Umberto's story, not only because it presages a 'miracle', but also to illustrate the important role of physical illness in the genesis of suicidal behaviour. Actually, there is a lot in this regard in Umberto's case, starting with his age, which is rather advanced. All over the world, elderly males have very high rates of suicide, especially if they are 80 or older. From 80 years of age onwards, elderly males have the highest suicide rates, be they from Australia or Italy or China or Uruguay. So, for most cultures, life becomes much more difficult for an ageing man than for a woman.

Physical illness also greatly contributes to increased suicide risk, again, especially in the aged, and especially in males. Potentially, all types of disease can be of concern, but in particular, when the disease process severely affects quality of life it creates dependency, constitutes a burden (financially, too) for children and other carers, and entails pain. Cancer can have all these characteristics, and causes great anxiety, especially in the early stages, as a suspected diagnosis has become a certainty. In such circumstances the resulting emotional turmoil and fear heightens risk. Disease or disability involving severe sensory deprivation (for example, impending blindness) can also be a major contributor to a suicide attempt.

However, the role of physical illness is greatly magnified by the presence of depression. A depressive disorder multiplies the risk directly associated with any medical condition. Umberto's salient comments reveal that after antidepressant treatment, the life-threatening and invalidating cancer acquires a totally different dimension and, if not tamed, is at least accepted, and then fought in a more appropriate way.

The relationship between Umberto and Tommaso, and their silent afternoons together looking out over the steeples of the cathedral — two old mates happy in each other's company — is a very lovely image. However, after Umberto's near-fatal suicide attempt, something changes in their bond and their communication becomes more overt and candid. Umberto's act seems to have eliminated the residual barriers to their interaction, and rendered their reciprocal positions more 'equal' and understood. Umberto does not like priests and psychiatrists; he considers them both representatives of unverifiable credos. Well, I am one of them (a psychiatrist), and I cannot but disagree with him. However, the message that I think we can pick up from Umberto's attitude is that, more than transcendental guidance, he was waiting for some tangible help, given by someone with a 'normal face' and warm enough to transmit much-needed human empathy. In the end, I believe this is what we all need.

And in fact, a few years ago the World Health Organization launched a slogan in this very direction: 'High Tech in High Touch' (high levels of technology in the context of a warm and empathetic medical relationship). As in any other socio-medical domains, the implementation of state-of-the-art protocols is necessary also in suicide prevention. However, this could not be enough to save a life. What is needed is to really care for our suicidal fellows, not just to make the 'appropriate' therapy. Even worse: suicidal persons have to be convinced that their carers are actually caring for them. This means that if this 'credibility test' is not passed for whatsoever reason, the care offered could be completely useless.

ELEVEN

In a Far Land

Maria's Story

aria is in a hospital bed, with catheters and a number of little tubes attached to her, but overall with her legs paralysed. This story was tape-recorded with her permission in the Geriatric Hospital of Padua.

Wine into vinaigrette

I am 73 years old. Old and tired, very tired. You can see what my condition is now. This is all my fault. God punished me for my weakness; He wanted to remind me that not everything can be done. Consequently, I am now just a paralysed elderly woman.

That tall and slim doctor with glasses (is he the director here?) told me that I have to accept my present situation, that I will never walk again, and that I am very lucky to still be alive. I should be happy then. He was not nasty but, you know, they tell you terrible truths with the tone of communicating that your wine has changed to vinegar. I cannot yet think about this story. Tomorrow we'll see; for now I just want to rest. I really would like to stop thinking.

It is my daughters who make me think of it. They now look in despair much more than me. I am sure they think that I am destined to become a big burden for them. And I don't want to be like that. I'll find the right place to stay, I am sure about that. I have enough money ... I'll find a solution. But not now, I don't want to think about anything now.

No, please, don't go away. I don't have anything else to do here, and they told me that it is days before you would have returned. Please, stay. My brain still works, and I can talk about everything. It is my body that looks like a battlefield; my head is working fine. This is why I think that God wanted to punish me. Otherwise he could have rendered me silly and lost, with what I have done.

You are here to learn my story, aren't you? They told me you are one of those who are interested in these facts. But, tell me, how is it possible to truly understand something if you haven't tried it? Or, have you? No ... In any case you wouldn't tell me, would you?

I have to tell you that I have known many psychiatrists and psychologists in my lifetime. When I was living in Argentina, I was analysed for 10 years by a famous psychoanalyst. Useful? Well, I could have bought a big house with all that money. Maybe even founded a big company. All those pesos for chatting — it didn't really help.

At the beginning
Do you want me to start at the very beginning? Well, I'll start from the first episode of my illness. Is this OK with you? I was 23 or 24 then. I had just arrived in Argentina. It was immediately after my wedding. My husband was the son of immigrants who made a fortune there. We met here in Italy, a year before, and it was love at first sight. When Hitler started his crazy war in 1939, my fiance asked me to go to Argentina to marry him. And so I did. I left everything and everybody here, and I took the ship. I got sick soon after my honeymoon. It was probably due to the incredible series of emotions: the big decision to leave quickly, my family opposing it, the war that was to commence, the long trip

through the ocean. And then the hurried marriage, the new country, the new language.

I remember that I stopped sleeping and eating. It is strange — instead of feeling horrible from this, I suddenly felt very well, as I have never felt before in my life. But those around me were very concerned about me: they thought that I was ill, very ill. They wanted me to stay in the hospital, but of course I didn't want to go. Why put me in a hospital if I had never felt better than this? And what would happen to my marriage? Surely I would have lost the love of my husband. To be honest, apart from love, he was the only connection that I had in that part of the world. No one from my family was there for my wedding.

I started to feel depressed, very depressed, and I accepted the hospital admission. I could not understand what was happening to me. I had no reason for feeling that way. I remained in the hospital — a psychiatric hospital — for many months, nearly a year. I was depressed and I couldn't recover from it. I was convinced that my best choice would be to go back to Italy, that the love of my husband would be lost forever. But apparently he loved me anyway. I became pregnant and was discharged from the hospital. Nine months later I gave birth to Carlo. Carlito. We always called him Carlito. Then we had Annamaria, Antonio, and Laura — she is the lady sitting outside here right now, did you see her? She has always been very close to me, poor thing. She has lived through so many terrible experiences with me. She teaches art, and she is very good at it. She paints quite beautifully: our home walls are completely covered by her paintings. And her students are so fond of her and they pay her so many visits, you can't even imagine. She never married. She has always been too quiet, too serious, that woman. Alas.

Where were we? Yes, four children; I had all of them in within nine years, and I was always fine. Nobody could believe it. That bitch of my mother-in-law; she kept telling me that I was too weak, that I had to take extra care of myself because of that, and that I had to reserve my energy, since I could not deal with everything. But I was feeling fine, and it was cheap and easy in those days to find someone to help you both at home and with the children. And honestly, I really wanted to be able to manage my family and my house without any help from my husband's family.

I sent Carlito to the Italian school. He was very good, Carlito. The best of them all, both at school and at home. He was very diligent, sensitive, cheerful, and full of energy. We were a very nice family, you know? Everybody said that. And maybe people remembered my illness, but the way I was running my family was so good that they genuinely praised my efforts. It was the best period of my life. Indeed. But then my husband died suddenly, possibly from meningitis or encephalitis, they said. For a few days he was sick in bed with a very high fever; then he slipped into a coma and after two days he died. Who knows, with contemporary medicine he could have been rescued, but at that time, in that country …

And then …

I was approximately 35 years old, and my world had fallen apart for the second time. I had been consulting the psycho-analyst ever since Annamaria's birth and I kept going for two more years, then I couldn't handle it anymore. I waited for Carlito to finish his primary schooling and then returned to Italy with all of my children. I sold everything I could: house, land, and cattle. Everything. Of course, my mother-in-law tried to impede it. She wanted Carlito and Annamaria to stay there to finish their schooling. Once finished, they could come to Italy, should I still be there. As I said, I resisted for two more years, and then I left. I didn't really have any good reason to remain there. In addition, I could not stand my mother-in-law's behaviour anymore — she was very intrusive; she wanted to control any action and know everything that happened in my home. How could she depend on a crazy woman, who was still conferring any power in her life to a psychoanalyst? She was trying to do both good and bad in my life, and I could not bear it anymore.

I came back to Italy with a lot of money, but also with a lot of despair. My mother died the same year as my husband, and I could not attend her funeral. I felt terribly guilty about that, as you can imagine. Years before, one of my brothers had died in Russia during the war. As for the remaining family still living, I had my elderly father and my eldest sister, together in the old family house. My remaining brother with his wife and three children were in Rome. I also had a sister in a psychiatric ward, but this only became known to me after my return to Italy.

To invest the money, I bought a few apartments. I lived in one of them with my four children. In the summer of the same year I was admitted, for the first time, to an Italian hospital. I also received electroconvulsive therapy. They told me that I had stopped talking. I could stay still for hours, even with my head suspended over the cushion ... Hard to believe it.

Virginia, the sister who was taking care of my father, also took care of my children. A cousin from Pieve di Cadore came down to help, and eventually she stayed with us indefinitely. I went to the hospital many more times. Once I swallowed all the pills I could find. It seemed to me that I could not significantly improve my situation.

How many times I have told this story? I am the first to be bored by it, even if each time it is like a wound that burns and bleeds [Maria cries]. I am sorry. I am very tired now. Could you please pour me some water? It is over there, on the table? Thank you [her eyes closed, she seems to have fallen asleep].

* * *

[Day after] You must be a very impatient person! Yesterday I had simply shut my eyes for a moment. Actually, I felt the need to pray and you ran away!

So, would you like me to continue my story? Yes? Where did we stop yesterday? Did I tell you of my husband's death? Yes? Did I also tell you about Via Savona, where we lived after my return to Italy? Ah, my poor head — you get lost in here, believe me. That woman moaned all the night [her roommate].

I need to tell you about Carlito. Carlito has been a big, big pain for me. Carlito never settled down here in Italy. He finished high school here and then he insisted on going back to Argentina. He wanted to see his grandparents again and especially visit his old places over there. I should not have let him go. I had the distinct feeling that something bad would happen. It is true that he had not settled in here. He didn't make any new acquaintances, and he maintained that he felt like a foreigner. He complained that his classmates teased him, because of his funny accent, and he could not stand it any more. I should have listened to my mother in-law; she wanted him to stay in Argentina and she was right. It was very selfish, on my behalf, to have brought him here, he said. He began to spend most of his time in his bedroom. He even started avoiding his brothers and sisters. He successfully finished his schooling and I couldn't say no to his request.

He went back to Argentina and never came back again. An accident occurred during a hunting adventure with his uncles and his cousins and now Carlito remains there forever, buried in Argentina, like his father. [Laura, Maria's daughter and sister of Carlito, thinks that he committed suicide shortly after his return to Argentina.] Do you know that sometimes I think that Carlito is still alive, and they are keeping him hidden from me to impede his return to Italy? But then I think that Carlito would never do something like that to his mother. He loved me, and he would certainly run away if they had tried to force him to remain there.

Sometimes I dream about Carlito. Once I dreamt of him and my husband, riding together in the pampas. Carlito knew everything about horses and riding. He started riding when he was five years old, with a pony that my husband gave him. He could ride like a god, my Carlito. Now, he must be riding with his father somewhere in heaven, I am sure of that.

Also Antonio has gone, did I tell you that? Antonio could not handle it. Life, I mean. He was too sensitive, such a nice creature … should I have remained in Argentina? What do you think? Antonio also complained a lot about being here. Poetry was his great hobby, but he wrote in Spanish. Poor thing, with a mother in and out of hospitals, and his brother dead in a foreign country. He thought that the Italian people around him didn't really want to understand him: he could understand everything in the Italian language, how was it possible, he said, that they could not understand him!

Antonio also fell sick, just before finishing high school. Some doctors said he was schizophrenic, others said he was manic. That is why he broke everything at home. Antonio had been so gentle and caring of everybody and everything. I think he could not accept the death of Carlito; in any case, something terribly bad happened to him, and he became a totally different person. Even his sisters, whom he loved so much, could not live with him any more and they were obliged to go to their grandfather's home. Only Laura could bear to bring him some food, but even then not every day, because he was often really dangerous and had beaten her on a couple of occasions. So Laura started to leave the food at the door of our apartment. She was so scared of Antonio that she used to ring the doorbell and then run away as soon as possible, without waiting for any signs of life from him. Anyway, Antonio was finally brought to the hospital. He stayed there for a while and appeared to recover rather quickly, but then he rapidly relapsed and was in and out over a few months, somewhat like me. But the very moment he looked definitely well, he killed himself. He hanged himself in the garage. You know, another son lost in that horrible way and right when his doctor told me that he was fine!

What more could I say? I had the worst days of my life. How can a doctor, a psychiatrist, be so wrong? What should I have done? Sue the doctor? I thought it would not bring Antonio back to me — I really was not interested in it and, honestly, I had a very good impression of that doctor. He really looked very serious and dedicated. I can probably understand those situations now. But only now, I must admit. You have to know that with all my misfortunes I never ever seriously thought about dying — I mean, to commit suicide. Can you believe it? And you should know, now, how many terrible events I have had to face in my miserable life.

Well, to be perfectly honest, there were moments in which I considered taking more pills than prescribed. But then my thoughts were for my children, my remaining children, and to all those horrible situations that had already challenged their young lives, as happened in my older life. And so, I kept going.

Can one understand?

If you ask me what happened to me one month ago (how long ago did it actually happen? I couldn't say ... what date is today?), I cannot explain. I really don't know how to answer. You see, I've always had great faith in God. An immense love for God, who always supported and guided me throughout my life. Otherwise, I would not make it, you know.

Please, think about it for a moment: my disease, which never heals; the deaths of my husband and Carlito; my dramatic return to Italy; Antonio's suicide; don't you think that is enough? And look: in all my life I had only that moment of numbness, of weakness; don't consider my madness — this was a disease and not a weakness of character. But for that single weakness, for that only moment, well, I didn't escape it. One cannot throw away one's own life, only God may decide upon a life. We cannot substitute Him in that, don't you think? My Antonio, he was sick, very sick. God will forgive him, I am sure of it. For what concerns me, hereinafter I'll always carry a cross that I have made with my own hands.

Maybe one day I will fully understand what happened to me. A doctor told me that it would take time before being able to put together all the pieces and reconstruct the entire picture. But he was such a young doctor, how could he really understand? How can he understand an elderly woman and her miserable life? What does he know about life? Do you think that 30 to 35 years are enough to know what death means, what it is like to lose a husband or, worst of the worse, your children?

I am really sorry ... I didn't want to offend you, and I have nothing against you. But I am bothered by the fact that here, inside this hospital, everybody pretends to understand everything, and this is really unbearable. And this is not because I am arrogant or pretentious — what do you think I am? I am just a paralysed, elderly woman, what else? But I lived a lot and, overall, I've suffered a lot in my life. One cannot understand these things by reading books, you know? Especially when the person herself does not understand what happened.

You probably know these things already, correct? You have already heard my remarks from other people. I don't know why I did it [Maria jumped from a window of her apartment, on the second floor] and if someone would try to explain it to me, I would probably not believe it. The only thing that I remember is the tension that was devouring me, the incredible disquiet that I felt. I was confused; I could not clearly think about anything. I was sleeping very poorly, in those days, and I didn't want to become a burden to anybody. Physically I was quite good but mentally ... yes, I have to admit that I was a kind of continuous lamentation, bothering everybody, myself first.

My daughters have every right to be left out of this suffering ... they have their own lives, and they are satisfied with that ... I have always tried to manage everything by myself. I really don't know whether I wanted to die that day or not. I don't know, I don't think so. I didn't want to suffer any more. Yes, that is it: I did want to stop that tension, to put an end to that unbearable suffering. I am not sure if you really know what anxiety is, that particular anxiety. It is like a devil that bites you inside, that squeezes your lungs. You cannot breathe, you really cannot breathe.

I have stopped feeling that way, now. It is true: I have lost my legs. They are the legs of an old woman; they have already gone where they needed to go. Now they can stay still. I don't mind it. I made a very big mistake and I have to pay for it. I can understand and accept that. I hope that God may continue to help me. Maybe He will.

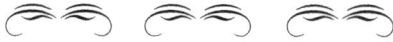

DIEGO'S COMMENTS ON MARIA'S STORY

Once more, we find bipolar disorder gaining the stage (other examples include 'A Busy Husband' and 'Country Living'). As with other mood disorders, this illness is strongly associated with suicide risk, normally more severe during depressive phases of the condition. With Maria's story, we are given no clues as to the appropriateness of previous therapies. We know that she underwent psychotherapy, and possibly psychoanalysis, but we have no information about the use of any pharmacotherapy, especially a mood stabiliser (such as lithium, valproic acid, and so on).

Maria presents with a number of additional risk factors for suicide. First of all, she had made at least one previous suicide attempt (overdosing with medication). A previous attempt is the strongest predictor of subsequent suicidal behaviour. In addition, as with Umberto (see Afternoons on the Verandah), she started to perceive herself as a burden for her daughters. In her life, the number of negative life events was simply overwhelming, with the migration to Argentina, the sudden death of her husband, her life as a single mother, and the suicides of both sons. Maria was a very stoic woman, managing a number of fundamentally challenging situations in the course of her difficult life.

Maria jumped from the second floor, a height of probably 7 to 8 metres; for an elderly person it was a very serious suicide attempt with the sequaelae of major spinal injury that left her paraplegic.

Maria's suicide attempt was probably unplanned. Her description of the moments preceding the act is instructive: she does not know if she really wanted to die; probably not. What she knows for sure is that she wanted to stop suffering, to escape from an unbearable situation, where her anxiety was 'like a devil that bites you inside, that squeezes your lungs'. Edwin Shneidman, an American psychologist considered to be the father of modern 'suicidology' (a term he coined), called this 'egression' — the desire to get rid of suffocating feelings and 'psychic pain'. Shneidman also explained that in many cases suicidal subjects do not want to die but rather to stop their psychic pain, the psychological suffering, something that perfectly applies to this elderly lady.

Now Maria seems quite accepting of the physical handicap following on from her suicidal act. She never again engaged in suicidal behaviour, as told to me by her daughter Laura, whom I met by chance a few years later. Maria finally left this life, aged 78, as a consequence of cardiovascular problems; in effect, dying naturally of old age.

Part
THREE

❦

Stories from those left behind

TWELVE

A Familiar Smell of Garlic
Diane's Story*

ear Diego,
Life is sometimes very unjust, as my story illustrates. What concerns me is that, even if I have received a lot, it feels like too much was stolen from me anyway. I am talking in terms of tranquillity, serenity, and inner peace.

Death in life

My mother, gold hair, eyes the colour of the sky, is always in my mind. Not too tall but slim, with a very elegant deportment despite her humble origin. She was very beautiful.

'Three and carry over the two, isn't it Mum? Isn't it Mum?' An intense smell of parsley and garlic, the rhythmic movement of the knife, and then nothing more. On a few occasions I found her unconscious on the floor, I always run for help, that damned door so difficult to open ...

I would never, ever come back and be a child again. Too much pain, too much suffering. I still have the scars on me.

Mum was finally found by one of our neighbours, a quiet lady who had helped us in many things before. She found her hanged in our cellar.

Even if many years have already passed, I still see in the face of my father the horrible pain of that moment. He

---

* Diane's real name has been changed to protect the privacy of the contributor.

doesn't say anything, but I can feel what he thinks. After 20 years he is torturing himself with what he could have said but didn't say.

After the suicide of Mum, an incredibly dark atmosphere took possession of our lives, smothering our smiles and rendering most of our days meaningless. There are children who permanently live behind their parents, whereas we have spent most of our time entrapped by the death of our mother.

When our relatives visited us, they embraced us, caressed us and kissed us. If someone external to the family were present, they told them that we are the daughters of their 'dead sister', and a special emphasis was given to the adjective 'dead'. Generally, a very detailed tale followed, using particulars and precise descriptions of 'where', 'when', and 'how' everything had happened.

But privately, apart from those public extenuations, heavy silences followed. In my life loneliness has been a very faithful companion. Loneliness and death is an unpredictable linkage, and deeply embedded in my life. We lost our mother and, in addition, we found these two companions always ready to remind us of their existence.

I can't really say that my life has ever been normal. Hearing all the time about that event made me believe that in life, death is always present. Of my childhood I remember an image that I saw in a storybook; it represented the traditional iconography of death, with a skeleton, a mantle and scythe. Well, for most of my life I felt that I had it behind my shoulders.

I have never been able to enjoy any present happiness, because I was always concerned with possible future misadventures (real or imaginary). I spent my days asking who could be next, since in life we are destined to lose first those whom we love most.

I am now 30 and am perennially looking for some stability. I often find myself looking at my mother's photo, searching for similarity, but in the meantime being scared by the possibility of resembling her in some way. She was beautiful, sparkling, and capable, but also terribly frail, insecure, and weak.

When I am depressed and teary, I pray to God to be helped to overcome those moments, and when I mistreat someone — overwhelmed by my strong feelings — I hope that this person may end my suffering by helping me to find some equilibrium.

Search for balance

The search for a good balance has been, so far, my reason for living. Unfortunately, my excessive sensitivity pushes me to live too intensively my emotions, and I am permanently committed to find some form of effective detachment strategy.

My classmate at high school knew me very well and also loved me a lot. She was normally able to pick up my bad moments and on those occasions, she used to say that my eyes became darker, the light of my face faded away, and my entire body bent as though my shoulders were carrying an enormous and very tangible weight. The oppressive load was so heavy it kept me confined to an armchair, paralysed and unable to get up for hours and hours. I often misinterpreted that inactivity for laziness, and felt deep feelings of guilt. When I was a little girl it angered me that I couldn't cry at all, not even during funerals, when we are entitled to cry. And I actually wanted to express my deep pain and suffering, but I couldn't — I simply could not. Overall, I could not cry for my mother. Very often I went to the cemetery, hoping to be able to cry at least in front of her grave. But the closer to her I was, the more difficult everything became.

Honestly, I don't think I have ever hated or blamed my mother for what she did. I literally could not accept that her dying that way was to cause our lives to so deeply deteriorate. And I am sure that what happened to my own existence also happened to the lives of my father and sister. For too many years our family has been a mess. We had to try to put the pieces back together, and mend a very badly damaged fabric: our family was nothing more, and if there was still love somewhere, certainly it was well hidden. Our roles of father and daughters were lost amidst indifference and intolerance of each other.

I believe that pain may be a powerful facilitator of your personal growth (and maybe this is so in my case). But what torture when it is too big and overwhelming! I really couldn't live my childhood or adolescence. I was too committed too soon becoming a good 'little lady', and too committed to my sister, for whom I was too old to be a peer and too young to be a substitute mother. When she ran from the house, they made me feel guilty for not raising her properly. I am sorry, but it was not my duty to raise her. This is very clear to me now, but at the time it seemed to me quite natural to accept that responsibility.

Suicide means death for those who commit it, but mutilation for those who survive. It is not a wound, but an actual mutilation, because what is taken away from us cannot be recuperated in any way.

Diego, still today, a good husband, a balanced life, and a supportive family environment are not sufficient to give me real serenity. Notwithstanding, one continues to live with ghosts, altars, and domestic beatification. The sorrow for me remains and will always remain. When this is due to suicide, beyond everything else, a profound sense of misfortune and sterility accompanies you.

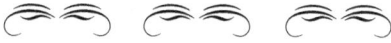

DIEGO'S COMMENTS ON DIANE'S STORY

This is a not-so-happy ending for Diane; it is is a sad story — the one left behind after their loved one has suicided. Sadly, given my profession, I have become used to the narratives of those survivors of a suicide death of their parent, children, relative, spouse, partner or dear friend. Such narratives are characterised by disbelief, resentment, insomnia, irritability, anxiety, depression, anger (towards the world, God, and the person who suicided), and feelings of guilt ('What could have been done?', 'Why I was unable to recognise the signals?' and many versions of 'If only ...'). Life for those left behind will never be the same. Equally painful is the stigmatisation by other people — the finger-pointing. When a suicide occurs the entire family is assumed to be 'contaminated', and its members treated as potentially 'infectious', as if they could spread dangerous suicide-inducing germs. In sum, extra suffering, because of the social environment and the culture, is added on top of the already unbearable burden of the loss.

This story has been included in this collection because of the lucid introspection of the protagonist and her 'paradigmatic' bereavement process. In particular, she is effective in calling her mother's loss a 'mutilation', because 'what is taken away ... cannot be recuperated in any way'.

She has reintegrated herself as best she can, completing her studies, marrying, and working in a job that she loves. However, this is a life lacking a 'limb', and she demonstrates an amputee's adaptation, as she says, like someone who has been deprived of an important part of him/herself. She can still achieve, but her life requires extra effort, extra resilience. Her legacy is that 'the sorrow remains and will always remain', together with 'a profound sense of misfortune and sterility'.

Suicide survivors often fear being unable to cope with the tragedy; they feel they might go crazy. Many themselves become shadowed by the dark compulsion of suicide — they may, especially around the anniversary of the death or birth of the deceased, or some other meaningful circumstances, attempt suicide themselves. Some consider themselves genetically predestined.

Evidence suggests that suicide does run in families; a product of genetic transmission but also of the family's 'script', the processes of psychological imitation (identification). It is still unclear what is actually 'inherited', though certainly for many mental disorders, a mechanism of genetic transmission has been demonstrated: depression, bipolar disorder, and schizophrenia are strongly associated with suicidal behaviour. Thus, an inherited mental disorder could act as a 'mediator' in the determinism of a suicide case. Also a 'given' are reduced serotonin levels — this essential neurotransmitter involved in the control of feelings and impulses is also associated with suicide proneness (particularly at the violent end of the spectrum), independently from mental disorders. A number of the genes implicated in the metabolism of serotonin could begin the genesis of such a tragic trajectory.

Recent investigation centres on a special area of the brain, the ventro–medial part of the prefrontal cortex (just above our eyebrows), which is specifically dedicated to controlling our powerful feelings by exerting appropriate inhibition on them. In essence, this area regulates our impulsiveness and, in part, our aggression. A reduced metabolism of serotonin in this area, genetically determined, renders individuals more prone to their strong emotions and to 'over-react' or 'short-circuit', with potentially catastrophic consequences, including suicide.

Research and clinical attention to the problems of those bereaved by suicide are both rather recent. It has only been since 1999 that the World Health Organization (WHO) included assistance to suicide survivors among their goals, via the SUPRE (SUicide PREvention) program (I am honoured to have contributed to that important initiative). A *WHO Guide for Survivors* was circulated worldwide in 2002, with an Australian (my good friend Raylee Taylor) providing the initial draft of the manuscript. An *Atlas of European Services* for suicide bereaved persons was published in 2003. Since then, much greater effort has been dedicated to this problem. In Australia, the Commonwealth and State Governments, and a number of non-government organisations (NGOs) have set up programs to support the (too many) persons bereaved by suicide around this country. However, I believe that this is just the beginning. Much more is required before the stigma that surrounds suicide and its survivors is eradicated, and before those bereaved by suicide become accepted and properly helped by our society.

THIRTEEN

≈ ≈

The Dream of a Life
Francesca's Story

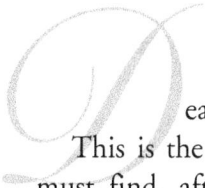

ear Diego,
This is the story of David and I, and how you can and must find, after a son's suicide, the way to redefine your world, the meaning of your life, and of his death. It is a story dedicated to all mothers of a son like my own, who left behind all his desperation, suffering, and defeat, and passed them to us in one action. We can be totally and absolutely shattered by that event, or we can try to transform it into a gift of love: it is up to us what to choose.

A survivor

I survived my son who committed suicide at the age of 17. I knew that I would be a survivor, before even knowing it, because I had dreamt it. I called it 'the dream of the Apocalypse', but I gave it a totally different interpretation when I dreamt it.

November 1991. My son is very low. He is depressed, bulimic, with crises of discomfort and aboulia. He is a very handsome boy. His face looks like a Norman prince, ancient and noble. When I look at him, I can see generations of ancestors emerging. Tough people, used to fighting warriors who came down from the north to conquer southern lands. Of those ancient fathers, my son has only the physical appearance, his body built with strength and elegance, but his inner part is fragile, delicate. His presence has always been impalpable and discrete, as if his brief passage was already in store.

He killed himself in March 1992, but he had been unwell at last since two years before that. He suffered from bulimia, even if at the beginning his crises were not very frequent. When I became aware of it, I contacted a psychiatrist, a friend of mine. I was very scared, even if I thought, in my ignorance, that bulimia is less dangerous than anorexia. Now I know that suicide is more common among bulimics. But the possibility that he could commit suicide never for an instant came into my mind. It was a fear that I never had.

At that time, my friend did not offer any help, or suggestion, or referral, although I told her that my son didn't do very well at school, that he was very secretive, and had few friends. He preferred to be by himself, and tended to avoid relationships with his peers. To her, all this seemed just an adolescent crisis. So she said to me, telling me what I hoped to be told: 'It is just his age, this moment will end soon'.

Then my son started playing rugby. And he was good, very good at it. He could show his character, had plenty of energy. The rugby league team for which he played kept an eye on him, and pampered him. His self-esteem grew and grew. Bulimic crises got less frequent. However, he was still self-contained and shy. His hobbies were of a solitary nature: fishing, philately. He didn't pass his school year.

He wanted to study agricultural sciences, especially because he loved animals, the earth, and plants. He had always been very fond of the natural. At age 10 he already knew the classifications of the animal realm, bird species, fish. He knew the name of every plant. He wanted to become a veterinarian too. His passions had always reassured me. I thought that his concrete, practical disposition would have helped him in life.

He was very aware of his own body, as all boys are. He put on weight around the age of nine, just three years after his father left the house and the family. This immature man assumed he had the right to live his life the way he wished, forgetting about his three children and then neglecting them completely since.

So, thanks to rugby, my son regained his physical form. He loved being elegant; he liked brand clothes. He spent hours in the bathtub, went often to the barber, and observed his muscles in the mirror. But isn't this what every boy does?

However, our family situation was very unhappy. At 33 I found myself alone, with three children to raise, without a job, no financial assets, and very little money. We lacked a male figure as a point of reference. In addition, in Italy, a woman with three children has serious difficulties in finding a stable partner.

I started teaching at school, and engaged myself in a long legal battle, frustrating and ignoble, with my ex-husband; a fight that, even after the death of my son, continued for many years. I am waiting for what is due to my children, something that their irresponsible father has always denied, not only financially, but also emotionally.

My son loved his father very much. He felt a painful nostalgia that devastated him. He never talked about him. If he did, he described him like a child that you need to understand and forgive. Clearly, he was not an ideal solid figure of reference. I froze once when my son said: 'I am my own father'.

A presentiment

I nearly always lived as a single woman, perennially struggling with financial difficulties, with very little help from my original family. I raised three children alone, unhappy and anxious about the future. I had my falls, my desperate moments, the constant fear of not being able to give my children the serenity and stability they needed. I felt many times powerless against the inevitable earthquakes of life, terrified of not being able to shield them enough from an unaffectionate and selfish father and from the many hardships of existence.

I had a presentiment of what was to come during the Friuli earthquake, in 1976.

My twin daughters were just two months old, and my son not even two years. I had just finished feeding them and put them to bed. I was going to sit down for dinner when that terrible shaking and roaring occurred. I had never experienced an earthquake before, and then I realised how vulnerable we may be, how precarious our condition. But then I didn't think of anything else and rushed like mad to pick my children up, in order to bring them out of the building. I grabbed my twin daughters in my arms and, like an automaton, went to pick up my son too.... And in that moment I realised something shocking, that was both terrifying and obvious, and that made me lose my breastmilk: I had three children and two arms, and I could not save them all. With what happened later, this was nearly a prophetic sign.

November 1991: my son suffers a lot. He cannot play rugby any more because he strained the ligaments of his right knee and needs an operation. This situation results in a great anguish. His excess energy can't be expressed or focused any more. He experiences this event like a further defeat. He thinks he doesn't deserve to be loved. He feels that he is incapable and useless.

Around that time my son falls in love with a girl from his class, whom he idealises, but he lives this love tragically, with angst. He is insecure, jealous, he fears for everything. He does not understand himself and the girl; those fluctuating feelings overwhelm him. He lives through them as if it were the first and last time in his life. Which will later turn out to be damned true ...

In this paralysing situation, bulimia grabs him again, and very violently this time. For a few months he went to see a psychologist. This made me feel a bit more relaxed, even if I was tormented by my usual troubles, frustrated by the never-ending legal battles, concerned with financial difficulties, and embittered by the loneliness that was around us. We have been left completely alone, my children and I, in the calvary that preceded the death of my son. The house, the walls — everything oozed with despair and pain.

Meanwhile, for a few months a violent sense of anguish was suffocating me. I had the feeling that something was going to happen. I felt it; I could even touch it. I knew that I was falling quickly towards a pitfall, but I didn't know why, nor did I know what could have been the black monster that was waiting for me at its bottom.

One day, exactly one month before my son's death, I wrote: 'Now it is the time. All my life I have tried to be ready for this; I cannot run away nor escape now.' I was aware of that. But I wasn't certainly thinking of my children. The tragedy was that this presentiment was getting stronger and stronger, clearer and clearer, but was still indefinable, even if I perceived it as unavoidable. What? What was going to happen to us? I then had the following dream, as clear, vivid and tangible as of a vision.

The dream of the Apocalypse

I was in a very brightly lit room, full of sun and colours. There was a conjugal bed, with the quilt of my parents that is now mine. The room opened onto a terrace, which faced a beautifully green plain. In the distance, there was the sea, blue and shining. Everything was beautiful, colourful, and full of life.

There were other women with me in the room. Suddenly, three small dots on the bed's pillow started to produce smoke, as if it was self-burning. I screamed, and in that very moment we heard a terrible roaring. We all ran outside and saw an immense column of fire and smoke, rising high in the sky. After that, everything disappeared, and I found myself transferred in a kind of 'day after' scene. All is grey; no colours. A sort of fog covers everything. The land is covered with ashes and wrecks. Indistinguishable figures are wandering in stillness; the air is grey, dense, and foggy. I can see my father (who died long ago) and my mother. My father is old and very ill, and my mother, while trying to reach for a gigantic pack of pasta, is crushed to the floor by it.

'Here we go', I said to myself, 'I am now alone; my parents are old and sick, I must manage by myself'. So I think that, if I want to start, I should pick up everything I can find and I start looking for a wheelbarrow to carry it all in.

Despite the dreadful surroundings, my state of mind is strangely serene and confident. I know what to do, I feel calm; I have only to solve practical problems. Where will I find a good, strong wheelbarrow? I notice a man and ask him if he can help me. He indicates to me a piece of cardboard, which is totally useless. Then I address myself to another man I spotted in the fog, but the result is the same. 'That's enough, I must handle it by myself,' I think, and look for, and finally find, a nice wheelbarrow, robust and well-kept. This special wheelbarrow is divided into two sections. I pick it up and I start to collect whatever I find; broken pieces, damaged glasses and cutlery. Every item that I collect gives me joy. At some stage, I think that if I went back, I could probably find things that I owned, relics of the house where I was at the moment of the explosion. So, pushing my wheelbarrow, walking over the ashes in that grey land, I decide to go back. But suddenly I am faced by a very high wall; across its top the following words are written: 'Keep out! Danger of death!'

'Gosh', I think, 'I'll quit my proposal; I'll find something else'. And I return to where I was coming from.

Now I can see a large road (which I hadn't seen before), long and straight, and I go along it, pushing my wheelbarrow. 'I want to go ahead. I am sure I'll find something, sooner or later.' In fact, at some point, I see a very huge store, with plenty of people who are partaking of food and other goods. So I fill my wheelbarrow with everything I think necessary. But then suddenly it comes to my mind that I don't have any money to pay for the things that I took. Nevertheless, with calm and confidence, I decide that I'll take what I need anyway, and then I'll see what to do about paying for it.

I was very impressed by this dream. I still am. The quality of the images was extremely vivid, different from usual dreams, as has happened to me with other premonitory dreams. Overall, there was a sense of serenity, of hope, of strength; all feelings that I missed in my real life at that time. In the dream I was a survivor, and now I know what it meant. Because this was the announcement of the death of my son and of what happened afterwards. Every single part of that dream, although expressed in a symbolic language, became true with impressive precision in the years to come.

The interpretation that I gave to the dream was that the shining and colourful world of my childhood, the idealised past in which I always took refuge in order to survive, was to be cancelled, reduced to ashes. I was growing up, I had to face my reality, which was surely grey and 'burnt', but I would have to deal with it with all my strength.

The three spots on the bed, I thought, represented my children. If I really wanted to help them, I had to say goodbye to the fantastic (but only in my mind) world of the past. I also must renounce relying on the idea of having parents, who were now unreliable and useless figures. Furthermore, the attempt to linger on my past constituted a deadly danger, as solemnly stated in the sign on the wall. I was very reassured by the concreteness and the peacefulness that pervaded all, my ability to take action and find the means to proceed and, most of all, the chance to find what I needed, without paying for everything with my blood, as it had happened until then. I had never had anything for free; nothing had been easy. From now on, it did not matter anymore: I would take what whatever I needed with great determination, and I would pay for it afterwards, not before. I should not wait for help from anyone, but expect support only from myself.

However, even if some part of the interpretation I gave then of the dream could still hold today, the full meaning tuned out to be totally different.

Shortly after that, my son had his operation. The intervention was very successful, and so was the recovery of his knee. But he needed a long rehabilitation, during which he had to remain still and rest a lot. Unfortunately, this was also the reason why his inner pain exploded. The suffering from his lack of ability to move, the overwhelming and uncontrolled energy, the fear that he would not be able to play rugby any more — everything fed his despair and his depression grew worse. He went from moments of total elation to moments of violent aggression, which was so very unnatural for his kind and sweet character. It was in these moments of aggression that I acknowledged the power of his despair and unhappiness. It was through this violence that it spoke its presence.

An inheritance

I survived for several reasons: I had to survive because I have two other children, because nature gave me very strong crutches and unexpected energies, and because my son left me an extraordinary inheritance.

I was very lucky. I spoke a lot with him; he left me a precious wealth of love and support. Especially in his last year of life, we spoke a lot, of him, of us, of things, and we said to each other, more or less openly, all the things that we needed to say and to know.

If nature had taken its course, and my son had lived longer, if he could have become an adult, maybe we would not have said any more than was already said. While leaving me, he offered me the key to his soul. Because this son, ever since he was inside me, a little embryo hidden in me, was really the son of my soul, the one with whom I had a secret and deep, strong connection. He would never become an adult, and his image will forever remain frozen in an eternal youth of beauty and pain.

Because of his knee, I took him to school, to therapies, or wherever he needed to go. This gave us more time for talking. And we understood each other very well. And this means, of course, that all this is not enough to stop a suicide, and if there is a depressive pathology or serious mood disorders, much more is needed than love and dialogue. These may be fundamental, but not necessarily sufficient. On the other hand, not even the psychologist expected that outcome, but it must be stressed that not all psychologists are educated or prepared to cope with every kind of emergency.

Now I know that all the warning signs were present. I know it now. And the suffering from being trapped in the impulses of bulimia was atrocious. He used to say that it was like a cancer, something he was unable to get rid of. In those moments of despair, in that complete isolation, in the absolute absence of anyone helping us, I felt desperately powerless to help the son I loved with all my soul. How I wanted to be able to rip out the nails that nailed him to his cross. But I was unable and could only carry it, together with him.

When we first openly talked about his bulimia, and tried to understand what it meant, from where it came, and how we could cope with it together, he said: 'I am finally relieved of a heavy load, Mum, now that you have discovered it. It is really a great relief.' But it was only a temporary relief. I did not know that there was someone in Padua who specialised in that pathology and also offered a public service.

The night before his death, he was studying Petrarch. I must add that the psychological therapy was starting to work. He showed some signs of improvement, he made some projects. I didn't know then that very often, when you see the first signs of remission, the danger of suicide is greater. Maybe it is because you can watch, in all its horror, at your sufferings, or maybe because that suffering, which filled you completely until that moment, is going away and is leaving an abyss of emptiness inside you, and this upsets you, and even shatters you deeply.

For more than one month he gave the impression of being distant. I now understand that it was like he had already said farewell to life. He wasn't interested in his stamps anymore; he observed his kitten with tenderness but didn't play with it anymore. He stayed many hours in bed. It was the most critical phase.

That last evening then, we talked about Petrarch and we laughed so much about him because Petrarch, I said to him, was a whiner. He always complained of everything. Had he, at least, committed this sin with Laura! He cried before the death of Laura; after the death of Laura, he always cried. He was an outstanding depressed guy, although a genius. How we laughed! My son had a great sense of humour and we shared this trait.

The next day, I drove him to school and then picked him up. Early in the afternoon, he was expected to go out with a friend.

I had cried all that morning: I felt scared, desperate, lost. I was thinking of my father, who died immediately after the birth of my son, and I didn't understand why I was feeling his presence so strongly. I desperately wanted to ask for help, but I didn't know how, where to, or from whom.

At lunch we had an argument over the scooter that he wanted to buy but had to wait for, and over other possible expenses, just money issues, very ordinary things in every family. He left the kitchen and went to his bedroom, shutting the door. I had the impulse to follow him, but I thought it was wise to leave him alone for a while, to meditate. Someone called me on the phone at that moment. As soon as I hung up, at five past three, one of his friends phoned asking for him. My son had been in his room for 25 minutes.

The nightmare

And now the nightmare starts. And never, ever, if they would have told me that my son would commit suicide, would I have thought that I would be here alive to tell his story.

I want to say what happened, because those who will read it, may also know that you can survive the total destruction of your world, of yourself.

I went to call him. I opened the door. He was not in. The room appeared completely empty. I didn't understand. I thought that he had gone out on the terrace, to smoke a cigarette. So I went to the window to see if he was there. Now, at a few centimetres from my face, I saw a 'thing' hanging flabbily. I didn't realise what it was. Then I 'saw' it. I thought that he wanted to play a terrible trick, as in the stripes of Dylan Dog, that he wanted me to read. I shook him, I called him, I shouted at him: 'Stupid, what are you doing?'.

I understand.

I split into two different beings. One starts screaming, to the point that her voice can't get out of her throat. She runs to the kitchen, to pick up a knife to cut the rope, she cries to her daughters to call a neighbour, the emergency line, an ambulance. She cries the name of her son.

The other, cold and detached, as in a dream thinks: 'How can I suffer so little for such a thing? How can I suffer so little in seeing my son this way? Why don't I drop dead?' She repeats these mute words while the other, screaming, is lying her son on the bed, praying him to come back, crying, trying to resuscitate him by performing mouth to mouth breathing. And screaming, crying, and screaming.

I thought my pain was inadequate, not normal, otherwise I surely would have died on the spot, killed by a stroke, or should become insane. Neither of these things happened. I don't know why.

The police, the ambulance, the resuscitation attempts — all those people rushing in and out of our house.

I was asked to leave the room: 'He cannot die,' I said to myself. 'He cannot die. Surely they will resuscitate him; they will come to tell me that he can make it. He was not born to die this way, at 17. This is unreal.'

The nurse of the Green Cross came to tell me that there was nothing they could do. I stopped crying, I stopped screaming. I froze, like a piece of stone. I sat down for hours. Still. While everybody was hustling around.

I didn't know what to do with myself. This was not the real world … In the real world in which you move, think, act, suffer, and speak. I was not doing any of these things.

I started wandering around my home, in total silence despite the many people, the policemen who were very gentle and really sensitive in handling the tragedy. One of them talked to me; he said that a few months before his wife had died of cancer and he understood me. He shook my hand. But I was looking at him as if he was talking in a foreign language. I perceived the sounds but not the meaning of those sounds.

People embraced me. But I could see no one, not even my daughters. It was like an hallucination. It was like walking, like being real, among the shadows of many ghosts. And, in any case, this was not reality. But which one was the reality? Now they would have come to tell me that they had made a mistake, that he was alive.

But this was not the case. They were not wrong. My son had died.

For three days I lived in a sort of limbo, with no wish to do anything. There was nothing to do. In the house there was a peace we never had before. A peace made of emptiness.

The tragedy for which I was preparing since my entire life, the one that for which I was awaiting in anguish, was here … That was it. What else could have happened to me? Problems? Nothing compared to this.

One thing was clear, from the very evening of that day. One thing, if still in a confused shape, waiting for further definition, but already clear in substance: I had to do something. His death should not prove useless, even if no death is such.

But the lesson, monstrous and atrocious, to be learned from his death, needed to be learned, so it could be transformed into life for other people.

I am not an ignorant or insensitive person; I had a good education, and I am able to connect with others, but I failed to understand what was happening to my son.

If such a young boy, kind and profound, who still has to discover everything in life, can choose to tear it away from himself, I had to help others before it was too late. They should not lack what I lacked: correct information and help.

But I was in desperation, and I was still living in another dimension. A part of me, the one that belonged to him, was with him, wherever he was. When you deeply love someone, a piece of you is inside that person. And if this person goes away, that piece is lost forever. It is not with you anymore. You don't own it anymore.

The moments I emerged from that sort of stony trance, I could only scream and cry. Everything was absurd and unreal. How was it possible that I couldn't touch him, hear him, see him, feel his smell anymore? Can a presence be there one moment and the next moment disappear totally?

I understood then what it means that a son's flesh is of your flesh. It means that you, with your blood, tissues and chromosomes, have made his mortal part, the material that contains his soul. And that is the one that dies, which is buried. With it, you are buried too.

I tried to remove from my mind the vision of his coffin disappearing under the earth and the dull sound of the shovelfuls of earth falling over the wood. But then I told myself that I had to let it surface and face it, if I wanted to get rid of it: 'I must do something. I must do something.'

Before, we were lonely and abandoned, and now our house was full of people all the time, the telephone was always ringing, the mailbox was always full with letters and messages. But what for?

There were those who felt guilty, those who we would never see again, those who were deeply moved and felt better human beings afterwards and more at peace with themselves. But there also were those who were sincerely sharing our pain, suffering with us and for us.

But all this meant nothing. Things remained the same, and it took a long time to understand the difference. And this happened to us too.

I was still a woman transformed into stone, and when I emerged from that stony dream, I could only cry and scream. Still, I was very concerned for my daughters, who also had to suffer all this.

Since then, our bond has become a very strong one.

A state of peace

Then, on the evening of the third day, something extraordinary happened. It was then that my life changed, that I changed. But, whatever happens, the suicide of a child cannot leave things unchanged. The world is not the same as before, you are not the same.

That evening I felt empty of life. I had no life before me — my life past. I tried to keep my hands engaged by knitting. I sat in front of the armchair where my boy used to sit watching TV.

Then, suddenly, I felt wrapped up, or embraced, in a sensation of inexpressible beauty, so great and wonderful, of peacefulness and bliss, which I had never experienced before in my life, and that could surely not belong to me, given what I was living through.

The grace of that feeling made me cry tears of thankfulness. It was a kind of fullness; I experienced a feeling of oneness with the universe. I was in harmony with everything. I was part of that harmony.

Buddhism has a special term to define this experience. There are no human words to express it, and I could only give it one explanation: my son wanted to let me know how he felt, and he literally had embraced me, wrapped me within himself. Since then, I feel a sense of peace I have never felt before, a strength, a clarity I have never possessed before.

Many times in my life, when looking for new ways to grow, for new paths, and to get rid of the dead weights, I tried to shed my old skin, to be born again. But every time I realised that I was walking along old and closed roads, that I was making the same old mistakes over and over again, with the same wrong behaviours. And consequently I went always back to the starting point.

Before my son's death, I had to acknowledge that all the possible new roads I could think of, all my attempts to change things, simply did not work. In the end, I always found myself in front of a tall wall, and I couldn't find the exit.

I did not have a clue what to do next. I knew I had to make changes, but how? That tragedy was the turning point and changed me for good.

That state of peace, of total detachment from things, lasted uninterrupted for months. I died with my son but through him, through his love, I was born again.

I gave him life, but he gave life to a new me.

I was slowly returning to the real world, from the distant and parallel world I went to the moment he died. I forced myself to perform every day a certain number of simple activities. I cleaned, cooked, bought groceries, put everything in order. I did everything very slowly, with no hurry. I needed to get used to this world through the eyes of the body again, since for many months I was not in this world. But reality had to be taken in drops, very carefully.

I asked for a leave from my teaching job. I was unable to be among young students; it was too much for me at that moment. In each of then I saw my son.

In the meantime, I was able to understand other people's sufferings more then I did before, and I felt compelled to console and support. Some people I met seemed quite scared to talk to me, because they thought they would have to face my pain and despair, and they went away full of peace and serenity.

But I didn't think that could be my permanent reaction. Or perhaps, I was slowly becoming mad. I was the first to doubt the nature of what I was feeling. Meanwhile, I strongly felt the need to transform the death of my son — this shattering event — into something useful for others. I needed to.

I discovered that in Padua there was the Italian Association for Suicide Prevention. I asked to meet you, Professor De Leo.

I must say that when I started to tell our story and said that I was there to ask for your help, not as a psychiatrist but as an expert, to hear and know what I had to say, you were quite surprised. Clearly, I was not a doctor, not even an expert, but only someone who had lost her son through suicide.

You didn't show it, but you remained speechless. Only later I understood why. Because usually total silence is what follows after a suicide. Family members do not talk, do not tell, often they feel ashamed, or they feel stigmatised in some way. My reaction was a bit atypical. But in this field, each person must find their own recipe for survival. One needs to give a meaning to death and a new sense to the remaining life. And I could see only one recipe to rescue my daughters and myself, to come out from horror through love. There was no other choice. Just to survive, or better, to live.

With his death, my son taught me such an immense lesson of love, and I can do nothing else but listen to him. What sort of a mother would I be, what sort of a person would I be, if I disregarded this precious gift?

It was not just for a selfish reason of my safety, it was a moral commitment, the duty that I took upon myself to go on being his mother, hopefully in a more adult and more worthy way. To honour him and his loving spirit.

He is and remains my son, even in death. I am not a practising Catholic, I don't like religions, because they are human structures, attempts to control the fear of death and of the unknown. But I've always had a profound sense of the sacred. And a great faith in God, whatever God is.

Since I was child, I felt that the entire universe is permeated by a harmony of which we are a part. It is our task to understand it and to conform to it through love. I say this because, if it weren't for my deep conviction, I would never have been able to survive. When I say 'after my son's death', I know that I feel much more at peace with everything; less angry for the injustice that I suffered, more able to understand and soothe others' pain. I started to learn how to love only since my son's death, and this asks for more love, because this was a sacrifice on the altar of our cruel times.

Learning to love is a very hard task. It requires strength and courage. And constant attention.

Life is a gift and a duty, but to help the living is also a duty, which implies alleviating others' pain. I feel, now more than ever, the weight of my imperfections, of my being selfish, the difficulty in getting rid of my limitations, and my tendency to always make the same mistakes. I tend to be presumptuous. But I must remember that I'm only human and that I am only a tool in what my son would like for me to do.

I don't think I could make it if I wasn't feeling his constant presence near me, especially that noble trait of his character, that made him understand other people's sorrows.

A new commitment

Throughout all my life I have been looking for fathers, guides, and teachers who would point to me the right path. I've found now both a father and my Master. He is my son.

Of course I would give my life to have him with me as a son, to see him grow up, make his own life, to become an adult.

But this is my reality, isn't it? The one with which I must cope. The one I must face. And I must take only this into account.

I was devastated by the pain he had to suffer, and how it grew to the point it did. If possible, it is this suffering that must be avoided in other young lives. It is also important to know that personality is one thing, and another is the effect of depression.

I would also like to help parents distraught by the suicide of their children, because I know what it is like to live with this unbearable weight until the end of your days. I also know that it would have been possible to rescue my son, if only I had had the right information, the right help. That is why I want to do something and say: 'There is nothing that will lessen your pain. You have to learn to live with it and to find good reasons to live. Even if life itself is a good motive to live, it may not look this way any more'.

My experience gave birth to the idea of creating an association for preventing youth suicide and helping parents who, like me, have lost their children. Putting together people who have experienced the same tragedy with experts in the field to support each other and study intervention strategies, particularly in the school environment, seemed to me the only possible answer. This is because there isn't much around, or very little, that may support families.

For years I have organised concerts, conferences, meetings, cultural events. This organising experience has proved useful in my new commitment. I agree: this is not essentially my life. I have made and I will make many mistakes. I have met and will meet many difficulties. This does not scare me: I have been through much bigger crises; I am used to sailing through stormy seas.

I have found a lot of sorrow around me, but also love, solidarity, and genuine interest. The net of solidarity is very rapid; it runs on a fast track, because there is an immense need for love around us. If you are willing to work, you soon realise how important this is. There is no point in remaining a prisoner of your pain, crying within a sterile suffering that cannot produce anything but poisonous fruits.

Despite the death of my son, the legal complications of my divorce, my financial difficulties, and especially my preoccupation with the wellbeing of my daughters, I can still see that there are many people around me who are far worse off. They have bigger and unsoluble misfortunes, they cannot find any peace, and they don't have any hope for the future. I was, and am, a very lucky person. Through a cruel lesson of love from my son, I was able to radically change an unacceptable reality. I found a new commitment for myself; maybe I'll become less selfish and proud. I am indebted to my son for what my life is today. That is why he is now my father. That is why I am his daughter.

The association is now growing; some institutions and many people are reaching out in generosity and human solidarity is supporting it. Not everyone so. There are also those who get lost on the road, because they thought they could use the suffering of others in order to get private benefit, for a launch trampoline. But this type of person is soon identified and left behind. Not with rage or resentment, because it's not to us to judge. But everyone must find his way.

Here and there I have my falls, my black moments, and I fear that nothing will happen, that everything will be very difficult, that I will not be strong or brave enough, that the association will never be effective. But I have learned to accept these moments, to live with and through them, because the pressure must be relieved somehow. I cry a bit, I get a bit down, but then I think that I am stupid, that I should not waste my time in that way. I pick up my rags and go on.

Sometimes I think that what I am doing may be out of guilt for not being able to help my son, for not understanding and fighting enough.

It could be. But even so, what's the point of wasting these precious energies now? These are luxuries that I cannot afford.

In my tragedy, I had the great gift of having my son with me for 17 years. I could have not had him. When I was pregnant, they were about to kill him, as the doctors thought that I had a cancer! And they were going to perform an operation. But it was not a womb cancer … It was my son!

His life is accomplished if, through his death, it will be possible to save some young people, to help a parent to find the lost peace and a new meaning to his life.

We need to go out from ourselves, look around in the world, with eyes lowered toward those who suffer like we do. These are obvious words. But so often in a man's heart the word 'obvious' does not exist.

Everything that is worthy and precious is paid for with pain and sorrow. Lasting conquests need to be earned, because life is sparing in treasures. But this is more reason for us to be generous, and we'll find help and solidarity especially by giving, instead of waiting to receive.

Thanks to my son, I understood these few simple things. It is terrible. But if expressing them will helps someone to understand sooner and better than I did, then it was worth it. I have found my main road, the one that was in my dream, which is leading me to the real nourishment.

Writing this story, which is a small part of my real itinerary, was a necessary step. On my journey as a wounded mother of a wounded son, I have met many other mothers who have found their children again through their death. With them we have talked, shared our experiences, and discovered that our children have a special language, in many cases similar, to make us feel their presence. None of these mothers are desperate anymore; nor am I.

The pain is there. It's always there and always will be. Time doesn't cure everything. But it can make the burden easier to carry. It emerges suddenly from time to time, when you don't expect it. A word, an image, a smell. But it is more bearable. It doesn't gnaw through your bones and flesh like it did.

To lose a child is an experience totally different from losing any other loved one, even if there is no healing in pain. A child is part of you, you made him or her, and they will always remain inside you. The light that this gave you, that life beside you, is now elsewhere. You don't know where. Not here, anyway. You cannot see your child, you cannot touch, nor smell him or her. When you try to close your arms around your child, they find a void.

It is through our senses that we perceive reality, and they are not satisfied. You discover that life is essentially this: contact. Touch. But you may come to perceive death in a different way.

I had already lost my father, and other people whom I loved deeply. With my son it has been totally different. Not only because of the traumatic circumstances concerning his death, but because I was his mother. I was his gate to this world. Finding other parents in similar conditions, sharing the pain and giving them comfort is a great gift, an unexpected relief.

This is the recipe

Do not spare yourself, forget the pain, and help others. Raise your eyes towards the holiness of existence and lower them towards the sorrow of others. Do not feel guilty. You did all you could. Probably it was not enough, but it was ALL you were able to do at that time ... and, in the name of your child, forgive others and yourself. Resentment, guilt and despair are powerful poisons; they kill life. They will kill you. If at the age of 17, enough despair can be experienced to reject life and commit suicide, this MUST teach us all something about humility and love, also for ourselves.

My life underwent a sudden turn, a total revolution. I also feel that the most cruel of evils may bring about some unexpected good. In an instant I became an adult, but I didn't lose the capacity to discover, to see the uncountable wonders of life. I was out from time and space, I saw the world like a two-dimensional, flat surface of nothingness, in which I did not belong. And then I came back.

I consider this part of my life as a mystical experience, like it is every experience that puts us in contact with the mystery of existence.

I understood what Dante felt when Beatrice died, even if the tie with her was so different. But what is described in the Vita Nova (The New Life) is exactly the experience of a death in love and of a new-birth in love. Dante had a pressing need to talk, to partake of his discovery. His voyage, at the beginning of suffering and then full of light, brings him to find Beatrice, an angelical being, as his guide. 'Donne ch'avete intelletto d'amore ...' ('Women, you who understand what is love ...') he addresses these women — such guides speak to you out of understanding, because (they) have already lived your own experience.

It is important to communicate this hope to all parents of a child who committed suicide, but who also died by other less obvious suicidal behaviours (often disguised suicides), like drug overdoses and road accidents. We should never remain closed in our pain. Our child would not want this.

Let's give to others the love that we would give to our children. It may be a way to give it also to ourselves, to heal the wounds in our soul. It is important to let hope feed us, because this is the core of mystery in every existence. Those who commit suicide deny, with their act, every hope, but also indicate very powerfully its enormous potential for operating good. This is the inheritance that our dear ones leave behind. How is it possible not to pick it up? How not to offer it to others?

The ancient Greeks had a specific term to express the concept of that experience, often traumatic, which changes your life through a revelation: 'chairos'. It is the unexpected, the intervention of fate, of the Gods, who with their terrible power subvert and destroy but also offer a way to resurrection. In one word: the revelation. They gave human form to this concept: that of a young boy of divine descent. This happened to me. Chairos, for me, has been my son.

Professor Diego, there is so much to do. There are so many people with plenty of generosity and willing to offer their support. Sometimes when talking with mothers, I find an unexpected energy from which to draw, and found I was able to provide some comfort in sharing their suffering. I found this in you, for you offered me your support and trust.

⌒⌒ ⌒⌒ ⌒⌒

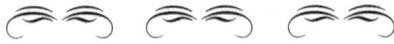

DIEGO'S COMMENTS ON FRANCESCA'S STORY

If a validating scale of human suffering existed, it would surely have the loss of children in its first position. Actually, in the literature there are examples of such measures, but the many variables that impact the score lessen any use they may have.

Parents of a child who has suicided know better than any scale can calibrate what losing a son or a daughter means to them. I deeply believe that the suffering from this tragedy is incomparable. Nevertheless, some of those parents have found new meaning in their existence by becoming activitists in suicide prevention. Francesca is one of them.

Francesca is a teacher of Italian literature. She writes beautifully. Her father was a famous scholar of ancient Greek literature; he left important work in this field. When I first met Francesca, she was directing all her energies into founding the Italian Association of Survivors of Suicided Children. She has since organised several conferences and gained recognition in national media.

There are many aspects of her tale that deserve specific comment, but one in particular needs special emphasis: her discovery of the body of her son. This appalling event carries the highest traumatic impact, and is usually associated with the onset of post-traumatic stress disorder, a frequent complication of such bereavement.

The 'splitting' that she perceives in her initial reaction to the discovery is also common to similar stories. She is surprised by her reaction: 'How can I suffer so little for such a thing?' — one part of her says this, while another part is convulsed in a silent scream. Francesca understands at that moment how even her present suffering will be nothing compared with the future anguish that will forever mark her life.

After a few days, she experiences 'total detachment from everything', which will last for many months. At this time, survivors should immediately be receiving help: they are in danger; their own life is at risk. They need to talk, to cry, to vent their despair, hopefully in a supportive environment. Loneliness or isolation can generate severe psychopathology, alcohol abuse, too many sleeping pills ... We can only guess what Francesca found in herself to be able to finally make it through, apart from being involved in many 'concrete activities'. It seems that she was resilient enough to manage by herself. Having to be there for her two young daughters surely had a role in her successful resurrection to a new, meaningful life. She quit her teaching job because she could not bear to be among young people any more; and in the meantime she felt a 'kind of transport toward others' suffering'.

In her account, Francesca effectively describes how she was able to understand, accept and transform the terrible pain from her son's suicide. 'With this death [he] taught me ... an immense lesson of love'. And this is what Francesca has now put into operation: her love for others. Not all survivors can find the same determination inside themselves, and even fewer are able to channel their residual energies into helping people facing similar tragedies.

You made it Francesca, and many are truly grateful for your support.

Epilogue

he moral of this book is, in essence, that we can all be resurrected, even from the most desperate situations. The human spirit surely has the ability to bounce back from the extreme lows; what we need is to remember this quality, especially in times when everything seems lost or irreversibly compromised.

The stories of *Turning Points*, with their unexpected but positive outcomes, teach us that it is within our capacity to find alternative solutions to existential crises and most dramatic situations, and that this is possible even when the world —our small world — appears to completely disintegrate around us. In those circumstances, all efforts seem in vain and all hopes vanish forever. But a Phoenix is actually there, ready to fly again for us. We have to keep this in mind. And in fact the stories tell us of the certain existence of the 'afterlife': not the one of religions (we might have hesitations about that), but the one shown by the many survivors who made this book possible. Those who survived the death of a parent or a child, and — overall — those who survived a very close encounter with their own death.

The reader will hopefully have identified many of the common risk-factors that contribute to suicide: psychiatric disorders, alcohol and drugs, sexual abuse, physical illness, losses, history of suicidal behaviours in family and peers, and so on. However, all these factors are also common to many other people who do not even consider suicide in the course of their lives. This observation seems to suggest that in a number of individuals there could be some type of predisposition, maybe a genetically determined proneness, as indicated by the well-known tendency of suicide to run in families (Ernest Hemingway's family counted five cases, including Ernest himself). Another explanation implies concomitance and 'piling up' of different factors; for example, being depressed, recently separated, abusing alcohol, becoming unemployed or perhaps physically impaired, certainly lower the threshold for suicidal behaviour, rendering it much more probable. Yet the vast majority of people would cope with all these misadventures, even if they happened all together at the same time.

We need the help of everyone to identify and provide timely intervention to those who may not be able to cope well and feel they cannot make it. In order to achieve this, we need more doctors and health services, better life conditions and more egalitarian societies, and so on. But — in particular — we need people more collectively 'connected', and more genuinely caring for each other.

We also need far more research than that which is presently funded. There are still too many mysterious aspects in the genesis and development of suicidal behaviours. More effort is needed at the biological, psychological, and social level, that will hopefully combine the complexities of these different perspectives and produce multidisciplinary approaches to the study of suicide. These approaches are possible, but they require more organisation and coordination than existing suicide prevention activities.

While the stories in this book contain personal experiences I have collected from people of two countries, Italy and Australia, I have also worked in other countries. However, most of my professional life has been spent in these two countries.

Italians and Australians (both great people!) belong to the so-called 'Western world', but are actually very different in many aspects: language, predominant religion, structure of society, diet, education curricula, governance and justice systems, currency, favourite sport, and so forth. And suicidal behaviour. In fact, just to add to the already innumerable complexities characterising suicide, culture and traditions are also extremely influential in affecting statistics and motives for suicidal behaviour. In the case of Italy and Australia, differences in statistics are more striking than those connected with motives. Suicide is twice as frequent (in relative numbers) in Australia than in Italy. And while suicide in Italy is more frequent among the elderly, in Australia the highest tribute is paid by young lives. To be more precise, in Italy a male aged 75 years or more dies by suicide five times more frequently than a young man aged 15 to 24; in Australia in 2005, men aged 25 to 34 have the highest rates of suicide. And while Australian youngsters die by suicide three times more frequently than their Italian peers, Italian elderly commit suicide nearly twice as frequently than Australian older adults.

Not many Australians live in Italy; *au contraire*, many Italians live in Australia. An intriguing aspect of their immigration is that rates of suicide in those of Italian origin or descent are nearly half those of Australians of Anglo-Saxon origin. This means that the rates in Australia are very similar to those of Italians living in Italy.

But why it is that so? Well, on this occasion I did not want to write a handbook of psychopathology, and here I wanted to be strong and avoid the temptation of a short course in suicidology. And I wanted to underline the enormous impact that cultural frameworks have on suicidal behaviours. As noted more than a century ago by Émile Durkheim (a French sociologist, still considered a key author in modern suicidology), there is no clear correlation across countries between rates of suicide and rates of mental disorders. This means that socio-environmental and cultural factors are more relevant than the prevalence of psychiatric conditions in explaining the differences existing internationally in suicide rates. As a consequence, suicide prevention practices should be tailored not only on the basis of age, gender and special life conditions, but also for cultural and ethnic origin.

A necessary, final warning: unfortunately, not all who survive a near-fatal attempt would change their life for the better. Those who regret not having died, or who keep going with their wish to die, and who even promise a more foolproof attempt at the next occasion — alas, they deserve our best attention. Their prognosis is not very good, and we are called to pay all possible efforts in trying to reverse their dangerous attitude towards death. This is imperative, since their risk of making a fatal suicide attempt will continue to be higher than the average population for many years.

Well, thank you for following us up to here. I hope that the stories in this book have given you the same sense of regeneration that they gave to me when I first knew of them and their protagonists. There are always other options in life: we have just to look for them!

Useful Addresses

www.auseinet.com

www.beyondblue.org.au

www.blackdoginstitute.org.au

www.burstingthebubble.com

www.compassionatefriendsvictoria.org.au

www.deleofundonlus.org

www.depressionnet.com.au

www.glcssa.org.au

www.grieflink.asn.au

www.griffith.edu.au/health/australian-institute-suicide-research-prevention

www.headspace.org.au

www.iasp.info

www.internationalacademyforsuicideresearch.org

www.indigenous.gov.au

www.justask.org.au

www.kidshelponline.com.au

www.lifeline.org.au

www.livingisforeveryone.com.au

www.menslineaus.org.au

www.mentalhealth.gov.au

www.mmha.org.au

www.moodgym.anu.edu.au

www.mulganet.net.au

www.psychology.org.au

www.ranzcp.org

www.reachout.com.au

www.readthesigns.com.au

www.ruralhealth.org.au

www.salvos.org.au

www.sane.org

www.suicidology.org

www.suicidpreventionaust.org

www.supportaftersuicide.org.au

www.who.int

Acknowledgments

My first thanks and *grazie* have to go to the exceptional people who, through the description of their dramatic experiences, have actually created this book. Umberto and Maria are no longer with us; they have passed away due to natural causes. Having known them was precious to me. I have learnt a lot from them, as I did from all the other contributors to this volume. Thank you indeed.

As in many situations in my life, this book would not have been possible without the love and incredible patience of my wife Cristina. She is a saint!

I am very grateful to James Cowan for his strong push to realise this work. His expert opinion was a powerful stimulation to me. I am also indebted to George Negus for his faith in my work and for convincing me of the potential interest of a general audience in these accounts. Perhaps his well-known passion for Italy has played some role in encouraging me!

Many thanks are due to Adriana Gagliardi and Jodie Bache-McLean, for their careful reading of the manuscript and for having helped me in the selection of the stories. Special gratitude goes to Julianne Schultz for her very substantial support and for having edited and published part of the Preamble in an issue of the Griffith Review ('Staying Alive'). Her splendid Mum, Cynthia Schultz, Honorary

Associate, LaTrobe University, has assisted by editing of the entire manuscript. Thank you so much, Cynthia!

I am also particularly grateful to Kerrie Eyers, for some valuable suggestions about structure.

I cannot forget the generous support of Jacinta Hawgood, my Deputy-Director at AISRAP, in trying to obviate my natural difficulties with the English language and helping with my translations from Italian.

I would love to thank (immensely) my son Vittorio for his typing of some of the stories, but this I cannot do anymore ...

Since I am apt to forget even my own name, I want to thank also all those who are not specifically mentioned here, but who have contributed to this book in some way.

You have helped to create a very worthwhile forum.